Psychosynthesis

Essays on the Theory and Practice of a Psychospiritual Psychology

Volume 2

Edited by Steve Simpson, Joan Evans and Roger Evans

Institute of Psychosynthesis, London, 2014

Published in 2014 by The Institute of Psychosynthesis
Institute of Psychosynthesis
65a Watford Way
London NW4 3AQ
UK

ISBN: 978-0-9572766-5-9

Design and typesetting by whosjack

Editor's Note

Welcome to Volume 2 of what we hope will now become a regular anthology of Essays on the Theory and Practice of a Psychospiritual Psychology, inspired by Roberto Assagioli's seminal ideas on Psychosynthesis.

Over the past 18 months, the Institute of Psychosynthesis London has been honoured to publish nearly 50 pieces of new writing, reflecting a wide and rich range of inspiration, ideas and application. Each article reflects a fresh drop in a deepening sea of consciousness.

As before, I want to offer heartfelt thanks to the authors of the papers contained in this book for their generosity and goodwill, expertise, insight, originality and imagination. As Editor, it has been a great pleasure and privilege for me to be one of the first to receive and read these varied but always fascinating offerings.

It has been said that psychosynthesis is a thought-form whose time has come. Certainly, our fractured, suffering world could benefit immensely from the insights and practices developed by Assagioli and those who have followed in his footsteps. In response to that need and the huge response to the call for contributions, The Institute of Psychosynthesis will continue to provide a platform for new writing on psychosynthesis and psychospiritual psychology. So, please, keep the manuscripts coming and I look forward to putting together a third volume over the coming year!

I hope, as practitioner or layperson, you will find something in the following pages synthetic thinking to inspire, provoke or simply evoke a sense of wonder.

Steve Simpson

Psychosynthesis

Foreword

In 2013, as part of the celebrations of our 40th anniversary, the Institute of Psychosynthesis published *Essays on the Theory and Practice of a Psychospiritual Psychology*, giving writers from the world-wide psychosynthesis and psychosprtitual communites a window to present their own experiences, discoveries and thinking. The intention was for this to be the first in a regular series of anthologies and I am therefore pleased to now welcome you to our second volume of essays.

Since 1980, the Institute of Psychosynthesis, London as a psychotherapy training Institute, has published a series of Monographs, annual Yearbooks, a Journal, and Training Manuals within a Psychospiritual Context. The purpose of these was to gather together a growing body of knowledge around a new psychology; one which recognises the reality of transpersonal experiences as being life-changing or meaning-giving events. As a discipline, psychosynthesis is engaged in the exploration of processes towards synthesis – whereby disparate elements learn to cooperate and work together to form larger and more unified wholes within the context of humanity's evolutionary journey.

Today, the differentiation between Psychospiritual Psychology and Transpersonal Psychology is much clearer. Psychospiritual psychology which is not polarised with transpersonal psychology is an attempt to add to it and move the debate on. The term has risen from within the transpersonal perspective and proposes levels which are not as yet clearly defined or 'mapped' – namely Spirit and Will. Anthony Sutich writing in the first Journal of Transpersonal Psychology said "transpersonal psychology is yet in its infancy"; even more so is psychospiritual psychology. At the same time, the term is not new to us. Assagioli himself in a series of lectures in Italy in 1966 used the term in a comparative study of some of the fields, particularly Jungian, akin to psychosynthesis. There he talks about dimensions of consciousness and the dynamics of the psychophysical, the psychological and the psychospiritual.

As the idea has developed we see that in transpersonal psychology there is a well defined personal and collective unconscious, and psychospiritual psychology adds the distinction of a spiritual consciousness – that of the Self. A psychospiritual psychology regards the Self as a reality, a living entity, direct and certain knowledge or awareness of which can be had. It recognises that the Self is a 'spiritual being' imbued with love which can be present to us in both its immanent and transcendent state. It mediates the interface between psyche and spirit and attempts to reconcile two fundamental experiences: the way in which we experience ourselves in our 'wholeness' – the way of spirit; and the way in which we experience our separateness – the way of psyche or soul, that aspect of Self which suffers separation.

Central to a psychospiritual perspective is the relationship between the 'I' and the Self. There is a marked distinction between consciousness, however transcendent, and the freedom to act in relation to just such a consciousness. The purpose of the process of individuation then has meaning beyond simply the realisation of Self. 'I am that I am' shifts the level of causality and brings with it an imperative to act in relation to that which one knows, making the 'I' an effective servant of the Self as it, at its own level, realises an ethical consciousness. A quest for healing or 'wholeness' therefore can be seen as a sacred quest towards becoming a moral being.

The essays in this volume are the wide-ranging. Whilst they do not all necessarily reflect the views and teaching of the Institute, they are welcomed as offering a rich tapestry of current thinking and practical application on psychosynthesis and psychospiritual psychology as it is expressed and practiced today, both in the UK and across the world. I hope these papers will be of interest and value to readers and inspire contributions to future editions of this series.

Joan Evans

Contents

Psychosynthesis as a Psychospiritual Psychology: an Evolving Idea

Systems, Synthesis and Group Dynamics

Joan Evans

From a still wider and more comprehensive point of view, universal life itself appears to us as a struggle between multiplicity and unity – a labor and an aspiration towards union. We seem to sense that – whether we conceive it as a divine being or as cosmic energy – the Spirit working upon and within all creation is shaping it into order, harmony, and beauty, uniting all beings with each other through links of love, achieving – slowly and silently, but powerfully and irresistibly – the Supreme Synthesis. (Assagioli, 1965)

Background

There is in the West what can be deemed a crisis of values in group relationships at many levels of organisation, whether they be within families, businesses, religious life, our education systems and more importantly internationally. With the world fast becoming smaller and our cities larger, the boundaries that are being traversed are complex and questions of identity and loyalty are being re-examined – for the most part in an unconscious and reactive way. For instance, someone growing up in England, can identify with being English and yet, at another level, know they are also a member of humanity. The consciousness of that other level seeks to be a living reality in my life. When the 'powers-that-be' organise the society in which I live by telling me that other members of humanity are my enemies, and legally create structures to reinforce that belief, I am inhibited from relating to my fellow human beings with love and compassion in a way which I believe to be immoral. As one growing up in South Africa, I had this experience as well as learning as the years have gone on that it is the quality of love that is empowering – the greater any group's capacity is for love, for forgiveness and for compassion the more able it is to express its power and its purpose. It required a leader with the spiritual consciousness of Mandela to able to transcend the splits within the nation. For him, every individual mattered regardless of race, colour or creed. In fact not only did they matter, but the national identity was dependent on the embrace of each and every one as part of that whole. His legacy to humanity was the power of his love which in itself transformed countless people's lives transcending differences which given their history had seemed impossible to reconcile.

This story continued for me about 30 years ago when we were involved in a group experience with other psychosynthesis practitioners. Our goal was service to humanity and the evolution of a life-giving psychology. However, the system was fiercely patriarchal and the rituals we participated in were not life-giving; they were against our own and other people's autonomy. We failed, and essentially we failed, I believe, because the individual was sacrificed for the group. The individual's right to structure his or her own life within the context of the group was not honoured. The individual's needs towards his or her personal autonomy were considered selfish and even against the group's purpose. The individual's contribution was generally judged as being not good enough, we were continually striving to be better than we were; different from how we were in an attempt to live up to some ideal unreachable image. An important lesson we learned was that the greater the purpose of the group – or in other words – the more inflated the vision, the greater the capacity is for delusion. Within that, individuals become 'possessed' or seduced by the vision and lose their discrimination.

On returning, after the group had literally turned in on itself and become destructive to its purpose, I began to wonder what the group phenomena was which had brought about such willfull harm. Naturally, this extends to political and social systems and I have spent much of my professional life working with and researching this very idea. I present here some of these ideas.

The Power of Systems

It is sometimes difficult to understand that the seeds for dynamics in the here-and-now have their roots in the past – and sometimes the ancient past. Physics tells us that there are 'initial conditions' which set in motion outcome and direction in any system. These conditions influence and impact on the field of consciousness as the system evolves. Unwittingly, therefore, we live our lives through the magnetic pull of the historical past which seems to have a will of its own despite our very best intentions. By understanding the system forces which keep us, members of the human family, impotent, disempowered and imprisoned in negative mindsets lie not outside of ourselves but deep within, not within any one individual or group, but deep in the unconscious field of which we are all a part.

Within the psychosynthesis world, the destructive and harmful elements of the 'group experience' are still not resolved and even though psychosynthesis has the context to synthesise the great contradictions, it, like many schools of psychology, are split into different factions. Even with all of our goodwill our commitment to service and understanding, the different schools find it difficult to speak to each other. Somehow, we are not able to transcend our history. The differences become splits and the other becomes the 'enemy' rather than the solution to the healing and evolution of the system.

These splits could have their roots even further back in the Cartesian separation between body and mind and the creation of dualism. There emerged the preeminence of the mind – that which could be seen, felt and therefore known. The deeper mysteries of the world of soul and the feminine became repressed.

The birth of psychology – the newest of the sciences – has as its context the ability to heal this split and to make whole that which has been separated. The great pioneers of the gateway into inner-space whose works described the pillars of this science, were Freud, the doctor, the scientist and Jung the Mystic and explorer of the deep unconscious which articulated very clearly the archetypes of Cartesian dualism; masculine and feminine, inner and outer, objective truth and inner knowing. Furthermore, if we were to peer into our ancient past it would be to look to the founder of psychosynthesis, Assagioli himself. His inner contradictions were to effect the development of the psychology he founded. On the one hand he was a scientist bound by rules of empirical study and on the other, he was a mystic with a profound interest in the healing arts, Thus, yet within his own psyche lay the seeds of a psychology of synthesis, reconciling the contradictions of science and mysticism.

Given the spirit of the times, he even went as far as 'erecting' a wall of silence between his own mystical journey into the unconscious and his explorations as a medical doctor and psychiatrist. This was in order to ensure his nascent ideas would be taken seriously within the context of empirical study. Perhaps it was this 'secretiveness' that contributed to psychosynthesis being so hidden in the years when it might have influenced more positively the development of modern psychology. And, perhaps it is this 'wall' that still prevents those of us from positively relating to each other. To attempt to resolve our differences at the level of group dynamics often fails and the status quo remains. Insight into what drives those dynamics at the level of the system is imperative. It is incumbent on us, in the psychosythesis world, to understand these initial conditions; to engage in a unified will to release them from the unconscious. Psychosynthesis is the Psychology that can transform modern psychology. It has the potential to be the voice that can offer the world a context and a ground for resolving such terrible conflicts, that exist now, politically, socially, ecologically and globally which are tearing us asunder.

The exploration of the nature of groups, their interpersonal dynamics and systems of which they are a part impact on the development of the individual, of society and of organisations. These principles have global implications and should be inherent in the study of psychology. Systems exist as substantial forms in the world comprising as little as three or four persons to many thousands. They have the power to overwhelm consciousness, to render individuals who inhabit or enter into their field to surrender their power, their thoughts and even their values. They have great power, with the capacity to move social groups to bend to their will, do harm and even disempower nation states. On the other hand, they are the most successful evolutionary structures on the planet which facilitate creativity, new thought beyond anything the individual could imagine or perform, as well as releasing individuals from the prisons of their history.

Synthesis and System Dynamics

Within our own psyche we are intrinsically story-tellers; telling the story of both our individual journey as well as that of our forebears – tribal, family and cultural as we function together in groups. This includes mindsets and belief systems of that history. We also see that we are the 'experiencers' of this journey that has unfolded through time where an idea that seeks to know itself, reveals and expresses itself through individuals and the groups of which they are a part. By articulating our experience we are able to access the unconscious 'system's forces' which affect group and team dynamics and most fundamentally our creativity in the here-and-now which the story and its 'history' may be limiting or even stifling.

To understand how this interplay and dynamic operates we can look at the work of Bohm (1980), and his theory of the implicate order. He describes clearly three dimensions of existence: the explicate order, the implicate order and a source of order beyond both. "The *explicate order* is a world of seemingly separate and isolated 'thing-events' in space and time. The *implicate order* is a realm in which all things and events are enfolded in a total wholeness and unity. The implicate order is not somehow inserted into material systems in space and time; rather, material systems and space and time themselves all 'unfold' from this underlying order." This universal flux Bohm calls the *holomovement*: 'This holomovement, which is 'life implicit', is the ground of both 'life explicit' and of 'inanimate matter', and this ground is what is primary, self-existent and universal. The holomovement 'carries the implicate order', and is an unbroken and undivided totality."' (Sheldrake on Bohm, 1988).

In other words, we come into relationship with levels of consciousness which are the consequence of our and other's experience of being in the world – both past and present. And in that sense, the world is not a given, rather we constitute our experience.

Thus there is the objective outer world comprising objects which can be seen, tasted and touched. We have internal mechanisms designed for us to synthesise the experiences coming into our senses and a 'common-sense' which makes

meaning of our experiences. This meaning-making function synthesises into a point of reference or belief system, which serves us surviving in the world.
There is also a subjective field or matrix which we know as 'consciousness' or matter, which is a dynamic interactive field always evolving. It creates and recreates itself in response to its own innate intelligence formed over time from the experience of individual selves being in time.

The point of tension between these two matrices lies at the heart of psychosynthesis psychology. That which seeks to emerge and that which has emerged and has become the 'stuff' of what we believe to be true. These truths or mindsets can often limit the emergence of anything new either in thought, belief or action. War and conflict rather than love and compassion for others are the result.

System Theory tells us that systems do not exist in a void (Lazlo, 1972). They interact with other systems. In addition to relationships on a 'horizontal' level, there are also 'vertical' connections, that is, a system is also part of a greater whole, which is a more inclusive system. Furthermore, a system itself is built up on sub-systems. The phenomenon of smaller systems being integrated with and harnessed by larger (more inclusive) systems is defined as a 'hierarchical organisation'.

System Forces

An organisation is a complex system which has developed over time with the individuals interacting within it. These interactions and the impact of the culture in which it finds itself gives the organisation an identity which includes levels of consciousness which have history, mindsets, ways of being and behaving in relationship to others both within and without the system. Going back to the 'initial conditions' of any organisation we find that these ways of being have been set in motion quite unconsciously.

Individuals can enter into the system at any point of its history and find these 'system forces' to which they are unwittingly subjected. Making these forces conscious allows for change and transformation and a greater degree of freedom for choice, cooperation and creativity. "The elements of a system have a high degree of autonomy and individuality on their own level. In other words, looking 'downward' the elements of a hierarchical organisation behave as complete within themselves. Looking 'upwards' they are sub-systems, subject to rules and laws, the blueprint and programme of the 'supra-system'" (De Vries, 1988).

The phenomenon of a system's integration with its sub-systems into a highly autonomous whole is represented by the concept of the 'holon', a term coined by Arthur Koestler (1975) to refer to that which is both a whole in one context and simultaneously part in another.

System Dynamics

Inherent in the psychology of psychosynthesis are principles which describe how complex forms evolve and devolve over time serving the emerging evolutionary thrust towards synthesis. This occurs as we attempt to create structures which would best reflect and transmit the ideas we are connecting to and which are a guiding force to our expression. In the late 1980s Eric Jantsch wrote extensively about self-organising systems whereby elements or forces, at their own level, create the tension for both the survival and transformation of the organism. Understanding these within a psychosynthesis context, has given us a perspective of both the world in which we are living and the psychology by which we live.

The four forces described below can be seen as system forces involved in the evolution of an organisation. Over time an understanding of the principles of empowerment, leadership and organisational structures emerges.

Koestler described two tendencies in this process, that of Self Adaption (SA) and that of the Integrative Tendency (IT). Ken Wilber (1995) has taken this concept further and points out that, "holons display four fundamental capacities; self-preservation, self-adaption, self transcendence, and self-dissolution".

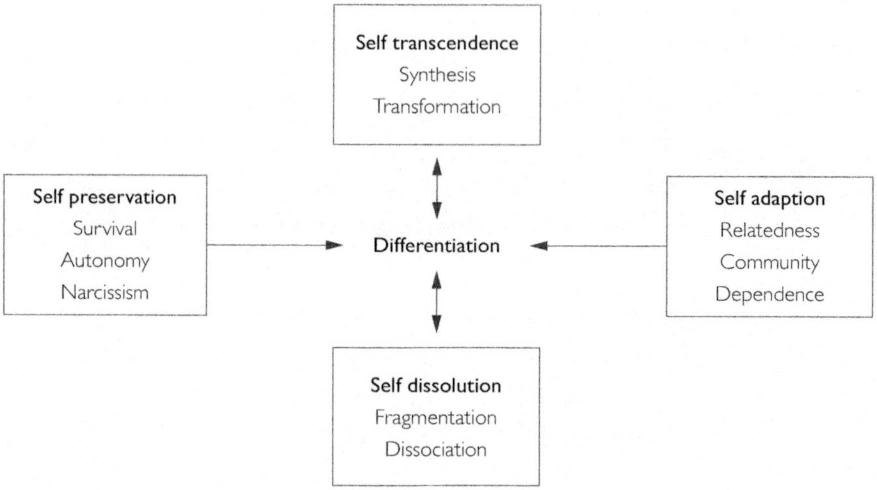

If there are swings too far either way along the horizontal axis we see the pathology of the system. There is breakdown, and dissociation or splitting off of the various elements and existential issues of identity and meaning emerge. Similarly, on the vertical axis, a system which is driven by fear or doubt may not engage in the risks vital to synthesis. To engage in transformation is an ongoing process representing points of reference in time along the way.

The Organising Principle

The intelligence of a system is predicated upon the relative availability of an organising principle which, in psychosynthesis terms, is seen as the Will around which the different elements cohere.

"...if we consider this process 'from within', we find that we can have a conscious existential experience of it. We can experience it as an intelligent energy, directed toward a definite aim, having a purpose. These are also the specific characteristics of the will as an expression of the synthesizing self" (Assagioli, 1973).

In order for there to be order and coherence, those elements which do not fit with the established order are repressed. If unintegrated, these 'forces;' build and eventually the system becomes unbalanced. The centre can no longer hold and chaos and fragmentation occur. In psychological terms, an eruption from the unconscious or unknown overwhelms consciousness, a period of darkness ensues and a new more complex sense of identity emerges.

This process of parts becoming wholes, occurs over time, as a principle of Synthesis. Paradoxically, breakdown in a system provides the fertile ground for the processes of integration.

"The differentiating processes are obviously necessary for the undeniable novelty and diversity created by evolution, but integration is just as crucial, converting manyness into oneness (the regime or canon or pattern of a holon is its integrative coherence). Thus Whitehead's view that the ultimate character pervading the universe is a drive toward the endless production of new syntheses" (Lowe, 1966).

Fields of Consciousness

For leaders at any level of an organisation, understanding group dynamics as well as system forces bring awareness to team processes and critical decisions that continuously need to be made. Exploring systems as they function prepersonally, interpersonally and transpersonally, we see that each describes a group mind or field of consciousness impacting on the individual's state of awareness and capacity for independent thought and action.

In looking at the group dynamics model described below, and drawing on Bohm's holomovement, we see that there are three dimensions driven by the principles of synthesis and which impact on the evolution of systems:

1 *Emotional Systems* are those in which an organisation's leaders contain anarchy as early unconscious survival issues are played out. Group or team members want structure and direction when psychological survival is at stake.

There are certain systems such as those in adolescent units, schools, therapeutic communities, impoverished social groups such as alcoholics or drug addicts or those who have been emotionally or physically abused which are served by wise and strong leadership who are able to withstand quite hostile energies as they find their way to their individuality. The leader is the 'tribal chief' – who psychically has the power of 'life and death' over them; who has the capacity to hold the whole and to generate life-giving processes. In larger organisations, they also have the capacity to hire and fire or to see they succeed or fail within organisations. On the other hand, there are powerful systems led by charismatic leaders who, by keeping group or team members dependent on them, maintain their own survival. These systems are cultish and extremely narcissistic eventually imploding and, often, becoming destructive to others as they, like a collapsing star, pull everything towards the centre.

2 *Closed Minded Systems* sit between the other two and are therefore pivotal points in themselves. They appear to be open and transparent, but sub-optimise towards the lowest common denominator. Over time, they cease to challenge themselves or to think out-of-the box and travel back and forth along the self-preservation and self-adaption axis of the 4-forces model.

Their value lies in serving the maturation of a system beyond survival and then confronting the unknown towards the next turn of the spiral. The power and wisdom of those steering or leading a system is crucial. It requires of them a willingness to let go to what they may not know; to be able to create an environment which empowers innovation and new thinking in a world for the future.

3 *Open Systems*. This is the goal and the context for the evolution of an organisation. Openness and transparency lie beyond fear and doubt and most importantly, beyond competition. At this level, the system is driven by cooperation between the parts, not only within the organisation, but with other organisations competing in the same field. It is emotionally difficult in a commercial world to see where the boundaries lie between where I am in competition and where I need to be cooperative.

For example as in the case of a Psychosynthesis Training Institute, its survival and the particular vision it serves needs to be valued and at the same time, to paraphrase Koestler (1975) it must serve the greater whole: "I am both a whole and a part at the same time. I am a London Psychosynthesis Training Institute; I am part of the movement of Psychosynthesis Psychology which itself is contextualized by the field of Psychospiritual Psychology. *I am, that I am*."

Group Dynamics

Group dynamics or the interaction of individuals impact on the system as a whole and are in fact the processes which give the momentum for it to evolve. Group work and team building are so critical because it is at the level of teams and small groups that change is determined at the global level and as such are the agencies for change within the larger and more complex organisation. "Think globally and act locally" (Schumacher, 1973), is the dictum for team building.

As early as 1965, Bruce Tuckman proposed a model for group development The Forming – Storming – Norming – Performing model described that "these phases are all necessary and inevitable in order for a team to grow, to face up to challenges, to tackle problems, to find solutions, to plan work, and to deliver results." Later in 1977 a fifth stage – Adjournment was added. In the 1980s William Schutz, an American Humanistic Psychologist developed a theory on Fundamental interpersonal relations orientation (FIRO) which mainly explains the interpersonal underworld of a small group. The theory is based on the belief that when people get together in a group, there are three main interpersonal needs they are looking to obtain: affection/openness, control and inclusion.

"The purpose of this work is to contribute to the development of more self-aware, open organizations and individuals with greater self-esteem. It is our desire that advancements in understanding the human element will at least match our advancements in technology. As we realize the tremendous power of truth, recognize our awesome capacity to determine our own lives, and overcome our fear of looking openly and honestly at ourselves, we can attain limitless heights of productivity and personal fulfilment in our organizations, our relationships, and ourselves" (Schutz, 1994).

Over the past 25 years, I have built on Schutz's work and developed a group dynamics model (Evans, 2007) taking into account work in the field leading to a deeper understanding of Systems and Synthesis. It helps leaders to stop, reflect and remember that there is a group dynamic process that they need to cooperate with and where appropriate facilitate.

The Group Dynamics Model

The following model describes the evolution and the group dynamics leading towards synthesis of a system. You will see that there are two fundamental processes on the one hand (the left hand side of the model) there is order and coherence. On the other (the right hand side) is chaos and disorder. Evolution cannot proceed without this momentum, particularly that of chaos and disorder. Team leaders need to be able to sustain and face these uncomfortable dynamics since greater consciousness and higher degrees of freedom to act are the imperatives for each turn of the spiral. Thus more intelligent and psychologically mature systems come into being.

As a system matures – over time – a field is formed which constrains as well as enables individuals' capacity to function freely within its boundaries. These boundary conditions determine their behaviour both interpersonally and intrapersonally impacting on their potential in the world. Taking into account group dynamics is crucial for organisational leaders in order to steer the organisation itself towards realising its vision.

This model can be applied to group work and team building as well as giving a perspective to whole systems.

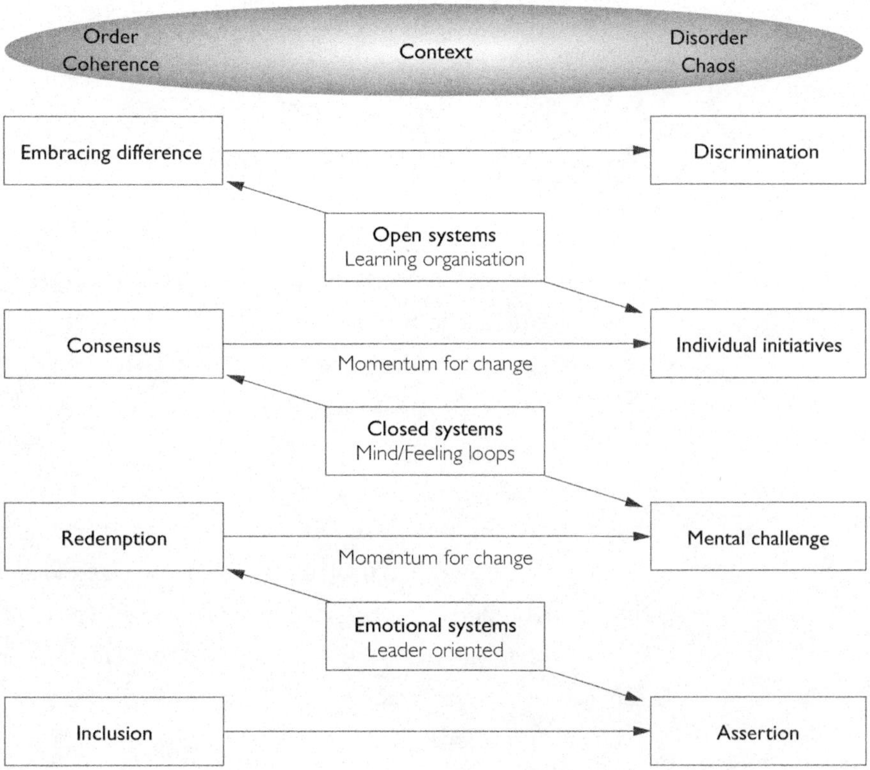

The Momentum for Change

Critical in the model are these pivotal points with the momentum for change. If the turning points are missed, denied or avoided, the group or team closes down and turns back on itself in a vicious cycle where eventually there is no growth or change. A group in this sense is unable to transcend its comfort zone even if the dynamics are unsafe and ultimately the organisation of which the group is a part becomes inert and uncreative and even unethical. For example, often it takes something of a revolution to effect the inevitable change which has happened recently in the commercial sectors, politics and the banking and insurance markets.

An awful lot of energy is required to maintain the status quo and the capacity for leaders to facilitate the confrontation with the comfort zone with care and compassion allows for growth and transcendence.

Emotional System Dynamics

Inclusion

The formation of a group or the start of a group coming together for an explicit purpose triggers certain dynamics based on history and story. These beginnings are therefore unique to the group, the place and the time given the different individuals whose stories converge at the formation. The family is the first group and its dynamics, beliefs and characteristics are projected onto a system whenever uncertainties of place, of power and of survival are considerations.

Initially the dynamics are largely emotional with trust and belonging issues being paramount. The capacity to think freely, out-of-the box and independently threaten the inclusion and belonging needs within the group. Emotional systems are leader-oriented, with the leader being invested with the power of 'life and death'. The individual's power is surrendered in order to belong with issues around survival being to the fore. The strength of belonging needs can be overwhelming with very primitive dynamics characterising behaviour. 'Follow the dictates, the belief systems and the tribal rules' leads to acceptance into and within the group. Quite unconsciously, in entering the space people begin to look for allies rather than those who threatens their survival. Primordial tribal instincts are at play: will I be accepted or thrown to the wolves?

Assertion (Kill the Leader)

Members in a group or team begin to explore their power in relation to the leader and each other. They are attempting to see whether or not they will have power as individuals within the system that they seek to be a part and ultimately have a voice in its ongoing creation.

The forms this takes can be fairly unsophisticated such as exploring whether or not it is acceptable to disagree with the group norms. This stage is still reactive and emotional in relation to the leader and his or her power. The power and will (Assagioli, 1972) is very important and over time needs to be embodied in each individual for empowerment to take place. At the pre-verbal level, the feelings, by asserting themselves, are trying to get a sense of the boundaries around the idea or the task. Assertion is not necessarily personal towards the leader, but in relation to what he or she is ostensibly standing for.

During this time allegiances are being formed and the status of the favoured son or daughter is being fought for. This is a difficult time emotionally in any group interaction. If rebelliousness and/or anger are repressed, a crucial dynamic towards a group's evolution can be lost. Although personally directed, it is important that a leader in this position does not take it personally but to absorb and allow the anger and tension of these dynamics so that the next stage can emerge successfully.

The Pivot Point and Momentum for Change

Redemption or resurrection:

Metaphorically, it is as if the warring kids come to the point where they redeem or resurrect 'father' in the form of the laws, rules and models of the group, which are then accepted as the way things are here.

To know that one is loved and that one can survive are the fundamental dictums for psychological health. Once there is a sense of trust in relation to these issues, and that the 'danger has passed', members are able to let go to listen to what the leader has to say, to honour what they have come for. As a leader it is important not to harbour resentment from hurt feelings or to have abdicated so completely that the group feels abandoned. There is now the acknowledgement of the leader and his or her authority and there is often more warmth and ease in the group. Once this step has been reached the group is then in a place to get to work effectively together.

Closed-Minded System Dynamics

Mental Challenge – Assertion at a Higher Turn of the Spiral

This may feel, and look like, more assertion, but it's important to see it on a mental level rather than emotional. It is about trying to unpack and get an idea clear. It is a mental challenge; not testing for power but reality in relation to 'truth'.

A system at this stage builds what I would call a mind, it can learn and its experiences can be evaluated. Space is needed to disagree, to have different points of view. If the leadership is identified with what they themselves are saying, it's going to be difficult. The group needs to think together, to look at what is true, rather than what they imagine to be true or what history has taught them is true.

Consensus – Communal Agreement

Finally, after the struggle, the group energy pulls towards consensus. Essentially, all members of the group get a piece of the pattern and they turn to each other to try and create unanimity. At any point an individual can connect to truth alone. At this stage truth is what the group thinks it is. Reality is created by consensus; they look to other group members for corroboration. Not so much leader-oriented, group members will talk to each other. The group is forming an articulated value system.

Many approaches that don't focus on individuality will stop here, and the consensus becomes the lowest common denominator. Group-Think is a term for this coined by social psychologist Janis Irving (1982): "It occurs when a group makes faulty decisions because group pressures lead to a deterioration of mental efficiency, reality testing, and moral judgment. Groups affected by groupthink ignore alternatives and tend to take irrational actions that dehumanise other groups. A group is especially vulnerable to groupthink when its members are similar in background, when the group is insulated from outside opinions, and when there are no clear rules for decision making."

If there really is to be a movement of the team opening up to the larger whole then the leader needs to allow the following to unfold.

The Pivot Point and Momentum for Change – Beyond Consensus

Individual initiatives:

Individuality is about standing alone with group members not being dependent on the group or the group's thoughtform for their survival – it Is OK for individuals to disagree with the group thoughtform that has emerged and go beyond it and in so doing take the group to another level of creativity. It is about moving out of the group mindset and beliefs and into values: 'What do I care about?' Individuals need to be willing to stand for their own voice as they conceive it to find their own way, to make their own mistakes or they will never go beyond right and wrong to a level of 'rightness'.

Apparent breakdown and conflict can characterise this stage and for the group not to pull back to consensus is imperative for the whole. The question is whether someone can stand up for their own voice and do that within a system openly and without fear of recrimination. Is the group psychologically mature enough to contain this? This is the psychological dynamic which provides the momentum for change. To keep trying to reach consensus is safe, but elicits a downturn rather than providing the impetus for the next turn of the spiral.

Open System Dynamics

To be able to be open and transparent, to risk unknowing and to be able to withstand uncertainty is a state beyond ego dynamics. The Dalai Lama has a concept of inner-disarmament which means living without fear and experiencing deep love and compassion for others – for all beings.

A system whose members live without judgement of each other, with appreciation and respect for other points of view enables a surrender and service to the 'greater good' and constantly living in the immediacy of the moment.

Embracing Difference and Discrimination

Allowing different points of view in the same space creates paradox leading to 'new thought'. This is beyond 'good or bad' or 'right and wrong'. It is about acknowledging that it may be different from the way any one individual sees it; and that any one can only see the truth partially. It is a willingness to include and honour differences. It is more than agreeing to disagree which would still be individuals holding on to their truth. It is an acknowledgement in the group that both it and the individuals in it are in service of something more than itself.

At this level individuals' inner experience resonates with their outer experience within the group and the group as a whole begins to connect to a larger context that it is serving. At the end of the day, the authority of the group rests in the idea; individuals aligned to that have as their indicator a resonance with their inner experience.

Conclusion

As an organisation of 40 years of continuous service, we, working within the Institute of Psychosynthesis, travelled all levels of the model and explored many aspects, the worst and best of systems and their dynamics; the worst and best of human nature caught in ego-dynamics despite laudable aspirations to the contrary; caught in history as well as rising to the spirit of synthesis and the evolving future.

It has been exciting to revisit this working model and to see that consciousness has grown and the principles of cooperation, of love and respect for those in this newest emerging psychology abound. It is a privilege to be a part of 'this greater whole' as we, with others, stumble towards the expression of its vision.

References

Assagioli, R, *Psychosynthesis*, Hobbs, Dorman & Co, 1965

Assagioli, R, *The Act of Will*, Viking Books, 1973

Bohm, D, *Wholeness and the Implicate Order*, Ark, 1980

De Vries, M, *The Redemption of the Intangible in Medicine*, Institute of Psychosynthesis, 1981

Evans, J, *The Awakening Self* (To be published)Evans, J, 'Group Dynamics' in *Psychosynthesis Psychology and its Professional Applications*, Institute of Psychosynthesis, 2007, Volume 6

Irving, JL, *Groupthink: Psychological Studies of Policy Decisions and Fiascoes*, Houghton Mifflin, 1982, 2nd edition

Jantsch, E, *The Self Organising Universe*, Pergamon (1980)

Koestler, A, *The Ghost in the Machine*, Picador, 1975

Lazlo, E, *Introduction to Systems Philosophy*, Harper, 1972

Lowe, V, *Understanding Whitehead*, John Hopkins Press, 1966

Schumacher, EF, *Small is Beautiful*, Blond & Briggs, 1973

Schutz, W, *The Human Element: Productivity, Self-Esteem and the Bottom Line*, Jossey-Bass, 1994

Tuckman, B, 'Developmental Sequence in Small Groups', *Psychological Bulletin*, 63 (6): 384-99, 1965 (Reprinted with permission in *Group Facilitation*, Spring 2001)

Wilber, K, *Sex, Ecology, Spirituality*, Shambhala, 1995

Reflections on Psychosynthesis: Self and World

Deryn Cooper, Robyn Rogers, Mark Skelding

A person is always in a social context...not an isolated unit...Deep peace...depends upon the harmonisation of wills...This same principle applies to an individual's relation to nature and the universe. No person can...consider [themselves] unrelated to the universe. Like it or not, (each) is a part of the universal will and must somehow tune in and willingly participate in the rhythms of universal life. (Roberto Assagioli, 1974, pp. 97-107)

Participatory knowing refers to a multidimensional access to reality that includes not only the intellectual knowing of the mind, but also the emotional and empathetic knowing of the heart, the sensual and somatic knowing of the body, the visionary and intuitive knowing of the soul, as well as any other way of knowing available to human beings. (Ferrer, 2002 p. 121)

If Self is defined as a singular noun, the planet is cooked. (Siegel, 2011)

The quotes above are relevant to the development of an experiential eco-psychosynthesis course, *Self and World,* in Aotearoa/New Zealand. Assagioli's invites us to awareness, Ferrer's addresses how we may access it, Siegel's encourages focus.

Self and World arose out of the experience, interests and training of three tutors of the Institute of Psychosynthesis New Zealand (IPNZ), founded by Helen Palmer and Peter Hubbard. Trained in the London Institute, for 24 years Helen and Peter have been developing psychosynthesis from a European-based transpersonal psychology into a psychospiritual psychology informed by the bi-cultural sensibilities of Aotearoa/New Zealand. This development aligns with the crucial recognition that psyche and spirit are of a wholeness which contains all levels of the personal, and the more than personal, dimensions.

Wholeness expresses in the middle ground, and therefore can be experienced in our daily lives – through the practice of Identification and Disidentification we can bring personal will into alignment with the ongoing manifestation of the Whole. In Assagioli's words: "At some point, perhaps in a crisis when danger threatens, an awakening occurs in which the individual discovers his will. This revelation that the self and the will are intimately connected can change a person's whole awareness of himself and the world" (1974, pp. 97-107).

Forty years on, crisis is massive. Climate change is just one of the symptoms of the systemic collapse we are living into. We are called to question personal and collective patterns, and consider where our world view, behaviours, purpose, meaning and values are failing. Assagioli, with his emphasis on the dynamic patterns of consciousness and will as functions of Self, has left psychosynthesis practitioners better equipped than many to explore and refine our own thinking and response to the call. Modern psychology has largely neglected the centrality of will, and has no place to consider the direct experience of Self, manifesting in the middle ground of our daily lives, albeit filtered and dimmed through the lens of personality, society, culture etc.

Self and World emphasises the experiential, following Assagioli's injunction that: "The right procedure is to postpone all intellectual discussions and theories on the subject, and begin by discovering the reality and the nature of the will through its direct existential experience" (1973, p. 6).

For him, human beings participate within Universal Will: "Let us recognize that if there was not a Universal Will, [humanity] would possess something not existing in the universe, and therefore the microcosm would be superior to the macrocosm – indeed a ridiculous conceit! The harmonization, communion, unification, and fusion of the two wills has been – and is – the deep aspiration and, one might say, the highest, even if often unrealized, need of humanity" (*Ibid*, p. 130).

In terms of Self-realisation, will, consciousness and awareness are inextricably entwined. Although it is impossible to conceive of will or consciousness alone, it is sadly commonplace for consciousness and will to escape awareness altogether. Body is the key. *Self and World* begins with body as the primary interface of self and world, an existential experience and expression of Will and Consciousness uniquely available at a distinct, yet not separate, point in the cosmos. We suggest to participants that Body makes possible a sense of place (location) and a sense of being (consciousness). Body is 'The Point of Existence' in Almaas's (1994) reflection on the inevitability of narcissism where Self is neglected or ignored (also see Plotkin (2008) for his conception of Western society as patho-adolescent), echoing Assagioli's "a ridiculous conceit". The result of the microcosm giving itself entitlements at the expense of the macrocosm is denial of our *physical* interrelationship, and exploitation of the systems on which we depend. This arises out of our physical, cultural and spiritual separation from 'will in action' and our failure to "tune in and willingly participate in the rhythms of universal life" (Keen, 1974).

Talking to a group of psychosynthesis practitioners meeting in London, Assagioli noted in Talks on the Self this separation from Universal Will: "This central fact of our existence and our experience, the most immediate, intimate awareness we have, is generally ignored or even denied. I could say, spiritually it is a scandal, but psychologically it is quite understandable, owing to the extroverted direction of Western Civilization, the final results we can observe all around us…The first thing is that each of us and as a group realize vividly the reality of the Self – because we are all mentally convinced of that or we would not be here!"

The language – 'realize vividly'…'most immediate, intimate awareness'…'each and as a group' – emphasises awareness as *physical experience*, personally and collectively. Such realisation Ferrer, Albareda and Romero argue, is immanent: "Perhaps as human beings gradually embody both the transcendent and immanent dimensions of the Mystery – a twofold incarnation, so to speak – we will realize that it is here, in this plane of concrete physical reality, that the cutting edge of spiritual transformation and evolution is taking place. For then the planet Earth may gradually turn into an Embodied Heaven, a unique place in the cosmos where beings can learn to express and receive embodied love in all its forms" (2004, p. 10).

Self and World examines how the currently transcendent times (the social thrust towards improvement – greater GDP, more consumption, personal development, self-reification, in contrast to Self-actualisation) ignore our immanent core:
"Turning and turning in the widening gyre
The falcon cannot hear the falconer;
Things fall apart; the centre cannot hold..." (WB Yeats)

Ignoring immanence opens up a gap in the flow of meaning, a split between individuals and ideas of fulfilment. That gap becomes occupied by mediators and regulators – priests, salespeople, even activists and psychosynthesists. Lacking the falconer, we encounter isolation, separation and Erysikthon's insatiable hunger (see Rust, 2014) where might have been transcendence. Death becomes a terrifying failure.

We explore theoretical understandings about consciousness, will and awareness. Communal, and grounded in immanent nature – both psychological and ecological – this exploration brings direct awareness of interconnected being, already whole, vividly reflected in the world and ourselves – points of vital experience and congruent expression – wherever we look. Anthropocentrism (microcosm/macrocosm misaligned) causes tensions between personal, transpersonal and universal will, resulting in systemic disharmony, disconnection, isolation, and atomisation (Assagioli 1973, p. 130). We present Plotkin (2008), Brown (personal communication; also this volume), Macy (1991) and Brown and Macy (1998) who see the tensions in the ecology of personal, transpersonal and universal will experienced, 'unconsciously', in crises of meaning, physical, emotional, psychological and spiritual confusions, and social distress. Each criticises modern psychology's anthropocentric illusion of separation, maintained when we assist clients to accommodate within the system causing their distress. Many clients leave then – the psychospiritual equivalent of the uncompleted antibiotics course; with symptoms alleviated, no deeper healing occurs. And as with antibiotics, resistance to the cure – cynicism and further separation – increases.

For *Self and World* employing IPNZ's modified Egg Diagram (Palmer, 2012, p. 49), with the Self star at top and bottom, the notion of 'unconsciousness' became problematic. To emphasise non-separation, we refer only to 'levels of consciousness'. Within the field of consciousness, personal centre of identity (PCI), our 'point of existence', is always at its unique moment – informed by history, biology, cosmology, culture, time and space. We discuss the meaning of the diagram as follows: awareness, poised between immanent Self-being and transcendent Self-becoming, expands and contracts within easily accessed 'middle consciousness'; basic consciousness in-forms and enables 'being-and-the-world' and superconscious inspires and transforms 'being-and-the-world'. Each shapes our experience, often beyond awareness, because of social, cultural or developmental constraints.

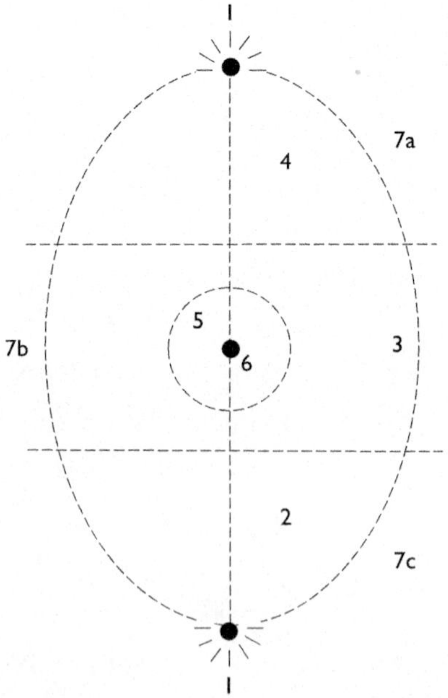

1. Self
2. Basic unconscious
3. Middle unconscious
4. Superconscious
5. The field of consciousness
6. Personal centre of identity
7a. Collective superconscious
7b. Collective middle unconscious
7c. Collective basic unconscious

Bringing in current understandings from neuropsychology, Siegel's (2011) description of mind – "a complex non-linear open system with emergent capacities for self-organisation" – fits Assagioli's model of psyche as a dynamic system, including participatory knowing and qualitative experience of all other beings (as subjects, not objects), and speaks to Fisher's suggestion (2013) that ecology and psychology are aspects of one system. Yeomans (1988) along with Firman and Gila (2002; 2010) describe interpersonal communion between levels of psyche. Using Siegel, Abram (1996) and Fisher we present this morphic connection as *psychospiritual* – intrapersonal, interpersonal, ecological, spiritual, universal – whilst attending to the *physical* restores Yeats' 'centre'.

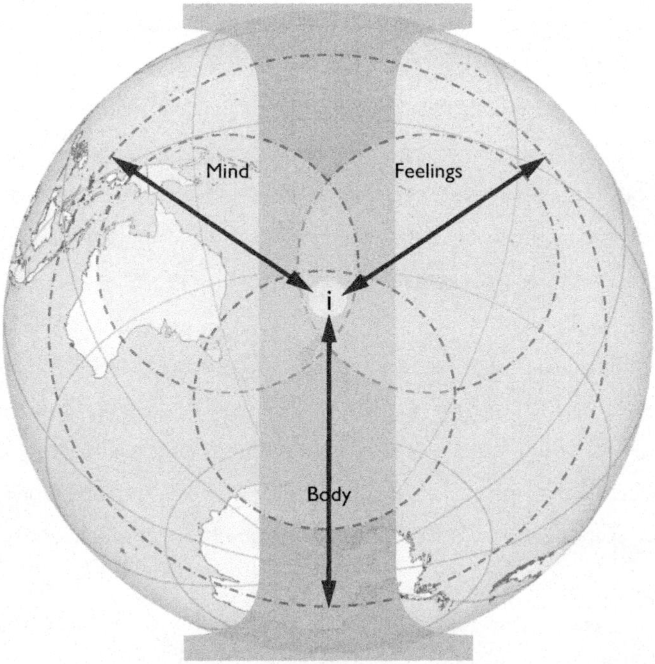

This second diagram is designed to show PCI expressing and experiencing through the BFM (Body, Feelings, Mind) matrix, with Self (grey 'I') behind, above, below and shining through, informing it, yet always more. In an anthropocentric view, building PCI increases our sense of capacity until whatever point (the wider circle) at which 'me' separates from 'other', 'we' from 'them', the Universe again resembles a collection of objects. Directing compassionate awareness to this complex nonlinear self-organising system – Body, Feelings, Mind, World and Self – builds PCI meaning-making and participation in the manifesting of will. Where many experience revelation, damnation, seduction or assault when self is ill-equipped to receive and process available information, participants hold the point of tension, and begin shifting from anthropocentricism to PCI awareness of Self at every level – the 'centre' holding, as personal, cultural and developmental insights ignite experience, and multiple points of view cohere.

To harmonise values and relationships, *Self and World* uses media, arts and science in ways that re-member rhythms of "the Long Now" (Brand, 1996) so alive in indigenous cultures including that of Aotearoa/NZ. Psychiatrist Mason Durie (Rangitane, Ngati Kauwhata and Ngati Raukawa) wrote: "The human condition is intimately connected to the wider domains of Rangi and Papa, the sky and earth parents [Maori cosmology]...health...is about harmonising people with their environments by actively promoting those indigenous values that have underpinned the human-environmental relationship over long periods of time...creating opportunities for people to experience that relationship first hand" (2011).

Avoiding colonising, or strip-mining indigenous cosmology, *Self and World* seeks contemporary forms – ecologian Thomas Berry, described humanity celebrating itself as a vital, healthy, connected element of the Universe, a new 'ecozoic' era where "...The primary principle of the Ecozoic is that the Universe – and in particular planet Earth – is a communionofsubjects, not a collection of objects" (1991).

As Ferrer suggested: "Human beings are – whether they know it or not – always participating in the self-disclosure of Spirit by virtue of their very existence. This participatory predicament is not only the ontological foundation of the other forms of participation but also the epistemic anchor of spiritual knowledge claims and the moral source of responsible action" (2012, p. 121).

And for quantum researchers, Hameroff and Penrose that "self-disclosure of Spirit" happens when "(t)he conscious moment and the quantum wave-function collapse are one and the same event" (2010, p. 52). For *Self and World* "the conscious moment" is engaged by directing awareness to embodied experience, felt as qualities, basic to the universe: "Roger (Penrose) and I proposed that maybe the qualia – the primary components of consciousness, of awareness, or at least their precursors – are also fundamental, irreducible, and built into the basic fabric of the universe. This could include Platonic information as well, such as the qualities of goodness, truth, and beauty. After all, why should the precursors to matter be present at that level but not the precursors to mind?" (Hameroff, 2010, p. 54). Assagioli considered such transpersonal qualities as basic. Psychosynthesis often explores qualities when considering how needs inform 'wants, behaviours, and world-views' – personality. *Self and World* also sees needs and qualities as immanent, prior to personality, basic to life and well-being, informing the life-force flowing between self and Self, *Self and World* – human distinctions of consciousness:

Conscious moment – Awareness of Needs – Experience/expression of Qualities – Quantum wave function collapse, participatory knowing and co-creation – "the basic fabric of the Universe" (*Self and World* model, 2014).

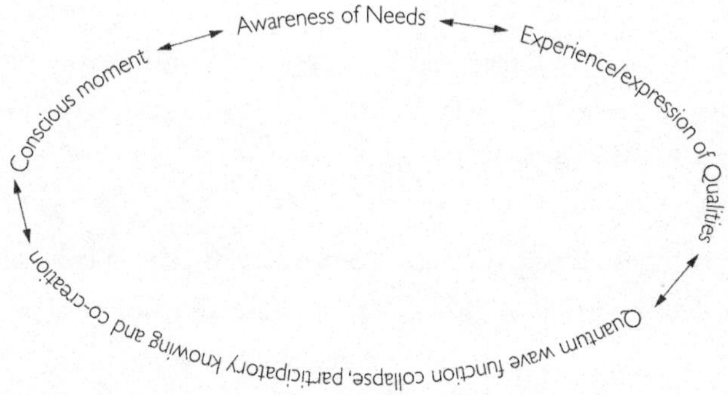

Recognising and responding in a qualitative relationship with our environment, via basic consciousness, places PCI in embodied service to the process: a tiny yet world-changing act of communion.

Hubbard also explored this phenomenon: "Schopenhauer the thinker and Assagioli the practitioner" concluding, "ultimately both hold to the ontological and experiential position, that 'I am Will'" (2013, p. 59).

Self and World seeks to link consciousness and will to the fabric of being and becoming. We draw on exciting and empowering knowledge unavailable to Assagioli, postulating how our direct qualitative experience may indeed link us to quantum reality. We remind ourselves that, for Assagioli, intellectual discussion and theory were secondary to direct experience – surely a call to engage Ferrer's "moral source of responsible action" (2012). *Self and World* supports participants to stand in the distress, pain and grief of our times, recognising our ongoing participation in these, healing separation, and opening to deep communion, as subjects, with place, planet and life – a sense of vitality, health and connectedness at all levels.

Through five weekends, spread over six months, the course invites a profound shift in s/Self alignment. Weekends begin with processes affirming the group physically (welcome, a shared meal, checking in) and *psychospiritually* (ritual, group meditation, shared meaning-making), grounded in the land and cosmology of AotearoaNZ, holding *tangata whenua* (indigenous culture) in respectful awareness, often presenced by our esteemed *kaumatua* (elder), Huru Te Manawanui Turner, 'PapaJoe'. Group-members build capacity and resilience exploring relationships and new meaning-making around familiar experiences and unfamiliar constructs, connected into the natural environment of West Auckland rain forest and beaches – a participatory ecology of Will-in-action.

Psychosynthesis elder, Thomas Yeomans (1988), championed a review of personal, transpersonal and spiritual dimensions as a psychological practice in the light of new ways of approaching the Mystery. *Self and World* pursues that review to face the challenges of our times, offering itself for people who wish to develop an I-Thou relationship with activism and the planet, without becoming psychosynthesis practitioners. The psychospiritual embrace of new scientific paradigms that affirm the universe as intelligent, purposive and seamless, allows celebration and participation in individual and collective wholeness, rather than definition by what we are not yet become. Siegel's uncompromising quote continues: "If we can find a way collectively that Self is a plural verb, to know that 'I am more than me, I am connected to you, and I am part of we', there can be different outcomes" (2011).

Beyond significant personal realisations, *Self and World* participants' outcomes included:

- Community art projects defining a protested ring road alongside a housing complex; renewal and deepening of commitment by a stay-home father to his daughters; translocation of a surf-loving counsellor from the city to a wild coastal environment
- Ecologically informed community education programmes
- Walkway on the family farm, with sculptures, ecological information, play spaces and sites for reflection where before there was no public access
- Development and promotion of the jurisprudence to enable those who suffer familial abuse to step up in service of healing a close relative rather than suffer in silence lest a significant figure be punished

Self and World addresses this: "An evolutionary response is being demanded that seems to require us to think in new ways. The challenge of change is to liberate more of our creative potential, engage the loving wisdom of our hearts, and express the highest sense of our values powerfully and in such a way that this response is made" (Institute of Psychosynthesis, New Zealand).

This revelation that…Self and…Will are intimately connected can change a person's whole awareness of himself and the world (Keen, 1974, pp. 97-107).

In memory of our beloved *kaumatua*, who died as we were writing this:
Huru Te Manawanui Turner (PapaJoe) (11 November 1930 – 5 March 2014)
Te aroha
Te whakapono
Me te rangimarie
Tatou tatou e
"May there be love, faith, and peace for all of us" (traditional Maori *waiata*).

References

Abrams, D, *The Spell of the Sensuous: Perception and Language in a More-Than-Human World*, Vintage Books, 1996

Almaas, A, *The Point of Existence: Transformations of Narcissism in Self-Realization*, Shambhala Publications, 1994

Assagioli, R, *Act of Will*, Penguin, 1973

Assagioli, R, 'Talks on the Self', *The Psychosynthesis and Education Trust*, London, undated handout

Berry, T, *The Ecozoic Era, Eleventh Annual EF Schumacher Lectures*, Massachusetts, New Economics Institute, 1991. Available from www.neweconomy.net/publications/lectures/berry/thomas/the-ecozoic-era

Brand, S. *The Long Now*. Available from www.longnow.org/about

Durie, M, 'An Indigenous Model of Health Promotion', *The Relationship Between Sustainable Environmental Practices and Positive Mental Health*, Mental Health Foundation, Auckland, NZ, 2011

Ferrer, JN, *Revisioning Transpersonal Theory: A Participatory Vision of Human Spirituality*, State University of New York, 2002

Ferrer, JN, Albareda RV and Romero, MT, 'Embodied Participation in the Mystery: Implications for the Individual, Interpersonal Relationships, and Society', *ReVision: A Journal of Consciousness and Transformation*, 2004, 27(1), 10-17. Available from www.estel.es/EmbodiedParticipationInTheMystery,%201espace.doc

Firman, J and Gila, A, *A Psychology of the Spirit*, State University of New York Press, 2002

Firman, J and Gila, A, *A Psychotherapy of Love*, State University of New York Press, 2010

Fisher, A, *Radical Ecopsychology: Psychology in the Service of Life*, State University of New York Press, 2013

Hameroff, S, 'Finding Spirit in the Fabric of Space & Time', *Enlightenednext*, 2010, Issue 46, pp. 48-57. Available from www.quantumconsciousness.org/documents/enlightenednext.pdf

IPNZ, Available from www.psychosynthesis.co.nz/introduction/

Keen, S, 'The Golden Mean of Roberto Assagioli', *Psychology Today,* 1974. Available from www.samkeen.com/interviews-by-sam/interviews-by-sam/the-golden-mean-of-roberto-assagioli

Macy, J, *World as Lover, World as Self: Courage for Global Justice and Ecological Renewal*, Parallax Press, 1991

Palmer, H, *Psychosynthesis in the South Pacific: Ontological and Epistemological Considerations in the Context of Aotearoa New Zealand*, Institute of Psychosynthesis, 2012, Monograph 10

Plotkin, B, *Nature and the Human Soul: Cultivating Wholeness and Community in a Fragmented World*, New World Library, 2008

Rust, M-J, Eros, *Animal and Earth*, lecture AUT Auckland, New Zealand, 23 January, 2014

Siegel, D, *The Neurological Basis of Behavior, the Mind, the Brain and Human Relationships*, Climate, Mind and Behaviour Symposium, Garrison Institute, New York, March, 2011. Available from www.youtube.com/watch?v=B7kBgaZLHaA

Wilber K, *Sex, Ecology and Spirituality*, Shambhala, 1995

Yeats, WB, 'The Second Coming', *Collected Poems*, 1989. Available from www.poemhunter.com/poem/the-second-coming

Yeomans, T, 'The Three Dimensions of Psychosynthesis' in *Readings in Psychosynthesis: Theory, Process & Practice*, Ontario Institute for Studies in Education, 1988, Vol 2, Eds, Weiser, J and Yeomans, T, pp. 243-253

On Earth as it is in Heaven: The Reluctant Incarnator and the Birthing of Spirit into Matter

Jessica Nelson

Psychosynthesis explores the human condition from the psychospiritual perspective of spirit incarnating in matter, a journey which involves risking potentially dangerous trials of womb and birth to arrive on earth. At each developmental stage of human life there is a metaphoric repetition of this birth cycle, separating from the known to be reborn in the new, in order to evolve to more complex levels of consciousness. To support healthy growth, the newborn needs to be safely anchored in the world.

The Institute of Psychosynthesis differentiates its concept of the Sacred Wound of incarnation from other psychologies of primal wounding. According to the Institute's model, existential dilemmas inherent in the Sacred Wound drive the soul's journey to experience and express spirit in matter.

We live in a dark valley, on a spectrum between the unconscious grace of the puppet and the fully conscious grace of the god. But the only way out of this impasse…is not back towards childhood: as with the Garden of Eden, an angel with a fiery sword guards the way…We have to go forward, through the travails and difficulties of life and embarrassment and doubt, and hope that…we may approach paradise again…and enter that grace which lies at the other end of the spectrum. (Philip Pullman from an interview with Kerry Friend, Amazon.com)

The novelist Kundera (1989) uses the phrase 'Unbearable Lightness of Being' to describe the deadness experienced by individuals cut off from the burden of feeling. Gaining weight, in psychosynthesis terms, can be understood as the identification of the 'I' with matter, a state which is a given for human survival in the early years but which can also be engaged with later in life as a conscious choice.

The 'I' seeks to express the qualities of Self through the vehicle of the human personality. At the beginning of its human manifestation, the 'I' undergoes successive identification with body, feelings and mind. This process throughout the developmental stages of human growth generates subpersonalities that interface with the outside world, ideally resulting in a personality strong yet flexible enough to convey Self.

The role of the 'I' in evolution of consciousness must first be understood through this necessary identification with matter, beginning with embodiment at conception. 'I' is the phenomenological experience of "being-in-the-world from the more essential experience of 'I' as the reflection or projection of Self in phenomenal awareness" (Assagioli, 1986, p. 19). A greater capacity for 'I' awareness thus requires not a way out of the world of human suffering but a deepening of the experience of spirit in matter, immersion in the territory of soul.

The aim of my paper is to explore the impact of very early trauma (from womb, through birth, up to the first few years), focusing on a certain type of client to whom I refer as the 'reluctant incarnator'. Many psychodynamic, object relations and Jungian writers provide a penetrating, empathic understanding of the earliest ego defences. Psychosynthesis, in its emphasis on bridging the realms of spirit and matter, provides a particularly coherent context for working with clients who suffer existential dilemmas at all levels.

Individuals who are fearful of life, on a constant existential edge of not wanting to 'be' in the world, can be described as 'reluctant incarnators'. My experience of working with such clients in my private practice is of encouraging the lost child to be 'born(e)' into the world, and to feel safe enough to 'bear' the weight of previously dissociated feelings. A thorough grounding in reality may help such individuals 'lighten up' by moving from an introverted withdrawal from the world towards realisation of Self, through true disidentification of the 'I' (rather than pathological dissociation, withdrawal or 'mystic flight').

Even then we are not talking about transcending the world and its realities, but of being in service to the world: "As soon as we lose contact with reality in order to follow the Absolute, we lose contact with the Absolute. The entire Absolute is contained in reality. There's not a trace of it elsewhere" (Devi, according to Daniel Odier, 1997, p. 85).

Guntrip (1968, p. 41), claims "the schizoid person at bottom feels overwhelmed by the external world and is in flight from it both inwards, and, as it were, backwards, to the safety of the womb". In psychosynthesis terms, this psychological retreat of the infant suffering early trauma impedes not only her ego development, but also resonates – like a fault line – at the levels of soul and spirit. Her ego cannot build upon a stable base because her sense of trust in a benign environment has been shaken. The innate human drive to differentiate consciousness may be hijacked by the infant's need to escape her pain in order to survive. In terms of her *psychospiritual* journey, flight from the world creates a dualistic illusion that Heaven is a separate place from the 'real world', and divinity external rather than an integral part of human 'being'.

Grof (1990) hypothesised that early traumatic experiences (Condensed Experience Systems or 'Coexes') could be identified at the core of each individual psyche, correlating with four corresponding stages of the birth process (Basic Perinatal Matrices, or BPMs):

- BPM I: symbiotic union
- BPM II: no exit
- BPM III: light at the end of the tunnel
- BPM IV: synthesis

Grof contended that a particular trauma suffered at any stage of the birth process would cause the developing ego to set up defensive patterns to protect against difficult feelings triggered by similar situations in later life. This results in the forward impetus of evolution becoming counteracted by a pull back towards imagined safety. In psychosynthesis terms, these two opposing forces correspond to the separate and distinct experiences of prepersonal will (at times *regressive*) and the expression of the Will of Self (*progressive*).

In conjunction with the Triphasic Model (Joan Evans, 1997), the BPMs describe how consciousness separates from an undifferentiated state of merger with the maternal matrix through to co-operation with the creative flow of the Universe. This journey of evolution requires the individual to cross a series of 'thresholds' in order to grow, each transition presenting an opportunity for spirit to identify with matter and experience human life more fully. Under the direction of Will the 'I', at appropriate stages of development, may loosen its identifications, allowing the individual psyche to become "harmonised and integrated in a *personal psychosynthesis*" (Assagioli, 1993, p. 55). Further potential exists for assimilation and integration of superconscious energies in a spiritual psychosynthesis.

Arrival

In the initial stages of ego growth, the infant's earliest experience of herself is of being at one with the maternal matrix. To the neonate, parents – with their power to transform hunger, cold and misery – are earthly gods who act as guardians of Self until the infant is old enough to rediscover her spiritual essence. In ideal circumstances, mother does her best to soothe the infant's anxieties arising from both her existential separation from the divine and her actual experience of the birth process.

Winnicott (1965, p. 52), claimed that for normal maturation of the ego, the infant required a 'good enough' facilitating environment: to be held both physically and emotionally, her emotions empathically mirrored. Persistent failures of the maternal care system may set up 'unthinkable anxiety' (p. 57) which fragments the developing ego.

A mother who is *unable* to soothe her child, as a result of her own dysfunction and that of earlier generations, will also have difficulty mirroring the child's divine essence or recognising any level of anxiety arising from birth and perceived separation from the divine. The infant, if not empathically mirrored at her most authentic – as a spiritual Self – by her environment, may encounter the terror of what Existential psychologists call 'non-being'. Not existing, in psychosynthesis terms, is an impossibility, since the Self is an ever-present ontological reality. Nevertheless, where the ego is underdeveloped, risking the metaphoric birth canal in order to grow in consciousness may seem more terrifying to the individual than the idea of death.

The terror of annihilation in the birth canal (BPM II) may result in a regressive pull to BPM I, the impulse to return to the 'oceanic oneness' of pre-consciousness, where 'bliss' emanates from merger rather than representing progression to BPM IV. This is consistent with Wilber's 'Pre-Trans Fallacy' theory (1996, Shambhala), which argues that evolution gets waylaid by the human longing to return to the Garden of Eden and a state of undifferentiated consciousness is mistaken for Heaven.

I have noticed in clients' stories a 'Garden of Eden' leit-motif, as though some memory of wholeness remains a blueprint in the psyche Clients may describe a 'happy' or uneventful childhood which they were reluctant to leave behind yet in which they remember no relationship with other humans; some talk of an internal 'secret garden'. I suggest that, in the absence of a safe enough early environment there may be a memory of oneness with Self which sustains the individual through traumatic events. This longing for a time, perhaps before birth, when a sense of well-being was last experienced, pervades the individual's psyche as an inability, or possible refusal, to incarnate – *in extremis*, as a longing for death – resulting in an ethereal, ungrounded existence.

One client, Lucy, was pronounced clinically dead at birth and had to be revived by doctors, living her early weeks in an incubator, unheld by her parents. When she first came to therapy, Lucy considered herself 'invisible'. The psychological environment colludes with this illusion: my reluctant incarnator clients are difficult to 'get hold of' in supervision and 'forgotten' between presentations; describe themselves as failing to get served in pubs, 'disappearing' or 'flying out of the window' when the going gets tough. Lucy said of herself, "I'm someone not even the cat takes notice of".

Each individual enters the world with a unique pattern of spiritual qualities. Innate personality traits may render some more sensitive than others to their environment. Eastcott (1980, p. 32), expanding on Assagioli's esoteric writings, suggests individuals assume the spiritual characteristics of particular energy rays as they incarnate. These attributes form the essential core of their personality, a theory which accords with Jung's (1971) definitions of differing personality types.

Whether such acute sensitivity precedes, or results from, early wounding, it seems clear that if the infant does *not* feel safe enough to trust either her environment or herself, there are obvious implications for her psychospiritual as well as ego development. Psychosynthesis differs from other therapies which work with the 'inner child' in that the repressed Child of Self (a 'Coex' encapsulating the nascent Self) is considered to possess the spiritual qualities with which the individual incarnated. Where there has been early trauma, the Child of Self goes into hiding as the Child of History (equating to Winnicott's adaptive False Self) takes over. The dynamics of splitting and repression thus explain how the burden of physicality and emotional authenticity may be shed.

Later Development

Psychodynamic and object relations theory suggests that the defence of withdrawal begins within the first few months of life. We know from developmental psychology that the capacity for rational thought does not develop in children until around the age of 7 years and the concrete mind may not be available as a defence until that point. If the infant who is unable to feel at home in the world does create her own place of safety and flies off there to take care of herself, we are left with the question of where exactly is this Neverland of the human psyche? Before we can encourage the lost child back into the world, we first need to know where to find her.

Reluctant incarnator clients often describe themselves as having been day-dreamers, their 'heads in a cloud' in childhood, suggesting that the only option available to a frightened baby may be to 'live' in the imagination, thus opening a gap between the child's *imagined* existence and outer reality. The infant has access to the imagination long before she has the mental capacity to make sense of her experience. In later years, when rational thought develops, the child may forge a paradoxical relationship with the concrete mind based on protecting her psychological place of safety, using her mind to keep her further out of relationship with life and other people. Johnson (1994, p. 25), for example, claims that to keep safe 'schizoid' individuals 'isolate thinking from feeling' to become 'mind-identified', tending to 'intellectualize' or 'spiritualize'. This defensive relationship with the mind forms the beginning of a maintaining cycle which continues to inhibit personal will: *I am safe so long as I do not exist; life is too dangerous and painful to bear, so I will not enter.*

Therapy with the Reluctant Incarnator

At each level of the Triphasic Model – Ego/I/Self – the dilemma for the reluctant incarnator is whether 'to be or not to be'. Working at ego level with clients whose prepersonal will is frozen through trauma is necessarily deep and sensitive, based on feelings and intuition rather than interpretation of remembered events. The reluctant incarnator often projects extreme levels of terror and anxiety which need to be held until the client has established enough ego strength to tolerate such disturbing feelings. The therapist must bear in mind the yearning for 'unborn-ness', which may underlie a client's presenting issues, sapping the will to exist. Experiencing safe holding, a client may be more willing to risk the metaphoric birth canal. Coming to therapy at all is a courageous first step; evidence of at least some willingness to participate in life.

One client, James, shunned human relationship and described his terror of 'falling backwards into an unbounded galaxy'. He spoke of a feeling he had on the point of waking every day, of 'slipping back into another realm', and the sickening recognition immediately afterwards that he was 'still in the real world'. Over a long period of therapy, James gradually 'settled' and became more relational, able to return my gaze. In one session, he connected to the part of him that wanted to regress to oblivion, feeling it poised on the edge of coming into life. I encouraged James to engage with this unborn part and the experience was of a descent of feelings into his physical body – which he had hitherto described as 'rigid and inflexible' – including grief for his own suffering and the first glimmer of self-compassion. Staying present to and recognising previously dissociated feelings in the body is a powerful therapeutic approach.

Once trust in the therapeutic alliance has been established, the depth work required to bring a lost child back to the world can begin. A child in hiding needs to be gently coaxed out into the open; encouraged to bring the jewel of the authentic Self into the world. Where early wounding has occurred, the experience of the core personality lies extremely close to the repressed memory of having once been connected to Self. When the Child of Self retreats at or around incarnation, the Child of History senses that her defences protect something sacred and precious, which if revealed to others may be trampled on. The therapist must exercise extreme caution around the lost child's terror of intimacy and intense shame. Paradoxically, an early lack of mirroring of the incarnated Self, may cause the client to fear being exposed as having nothing to offer. Here the therapist's task will be to witness the sense of uniqueness which was so seriously undermined.

In cases of profound soul trauma early in life, the internal world of the Child of Self may be hidden even from her adult self. When an individual has relied historically on the concrete mind to keep her safe, her emotions are tied up defending the ego from perceived external threats. Fear blocks her connection to the world of Self. In this way, the concrete mind begins to create a ceiling believing the individual to be nothing more than matter. The emphasis of therapy thus needs to be on whatever it takes to unhook the feelings from the mind's preoccupation with the perceived need to survive, freeing it to look up to the stars and contemplate spirit.

Working with media such as clay, free drawing or journal writing may serve to bypass the often harsh judgment of the concrete mind, whilst the Chakra model can provide a non-threatening and effective context for mirroring a tricky relationship with groundedness. Those in 'mystic flight' can relate without shame to a mirror which reflects that while they may be strong and fluent in the upper, more spiritual chakras (Ajna; Crown), there may be work to do around deficiencies in the base chakra, to secure stability in the world, or the solar plexus, in order to deepen relationship with the other.

The ability to open to the realm of the imagination may in time and with understanding become the means by which the reluctant incarnator returns to the world bearing precious gifts. Problems do arise, however, when – like Peter Pan – she is unable to return from her fantasy world. In order to come and go safely to and from the Neverland, the child needs a secure base and confidence that Mother will be there waiting with open arms when she returns.

The child's 'escape route' from the world may have established links to the imagination which bode well for her return from the Neverland. However, lack of mirroring of this imaginal facility may have left the client fearing that she is 'making things up', or that nothing is real. Some mistake the fantasy or mystic realm in which they take refuge for reality. The key may be to affirm and strengthen the client's relationship to imagination, which can be used for pragmatic purposes of grounding as well as to access the esoteric. Before every frightening meeting with another person, or worrying event, James first practices the encounter in the imagination, thereby making it possible for him to face in reality and taking some of the sting out of painful exposure. In employing this method, he engages Skillful Will to counteract the defensive accumulation of 'consciousness' that previously inhibited him.

Psychosynthesis regards imagination as the gateway into realms of consciousness at every level, allowing the individual access to all levels of the unconscious. Spirit is brought down from the abstract mind into the personality via the bridge of imagination. The abstract mind, the seat of intuition, is our link to both soul and spirit. The capacity to imagine something better or different and to bring that idea into reality is mankind's evolutionary tool.

Once reluctant incarnators' access to the imagination has been re-established, healing the trauma of early wounding at ego level can take place. Henry and Lucy were both eventually able to visualise and dialogue with subpersonalities. Henry, whose early defence of withdrawal had been triggered over and over in a repressive family, boarding school and armed forces background, described his first therapeutic encounter with his Child of Self as having the atmosphere of a séance, 'as though another presence had entered the room'. Over time, Henry's 'wild child' became very real to him, teaching him a lot he had 'forgotten' about his sensitivity, his compassion and his creativity.

Disconnected from the emotional content of suicide attempts earlier in her life, Lucy held me at arm's length until in one session I risked sharing the image of a young girl I was 'seeing', cowering in a corner. Lucy responded as though I had 'got' her, telling me all about the terrified child and what her impact had been on Lucy's adult life. Gradually, she was able to integrate emotions wrapped up in abandonment depression underlying suicidal thoughts.

At soul level, the longing for merger also manifests as 'Divine Homesickness;' a yearning to return to spirit. The therapist needs to watch for this level of suffering, bringing it to the client's awareness without trying to fix it. The client who has protected herself from early trauma through psychological flight will inevitably need to descend into the emotional as well as physical realm, learning through therapy to differentiate and tolerate a variety of emotions. The ground of soul is where clients begin to re-enter the 'real' world, taking up the burden of feelings they have left behind en route.

As therapy progressed, Henry began dreaming of a staircase leading deep into the ocean. He knew he needed to go down the staircase, but was afraid: visualisations helped to reassure him he had something to hold onto and could go at his own pace. On one of these occasions, Henry encountered a Wise Man (an aspect of his Higher Self) who was ready to accompany him as he made his descent.

In time, an individual's inner reality may be brought to life in service of reconnecting her to the values she considers worth living for. With patience and empathy – opening her own heart to Love and to the client – the therapist may eventually be granted entry to what Kelley-Lainé (1977, p. 102) calls the 'sacred tabernacle' of a client's psyche.

Sensitivity and creativity – whether innate, or resulting from early wounding – may be among the qualities the reluctant incarnator brings from her secret garden out into the world. 'Creating' allows the world to 'see' and share the internal world such clients find so difficult to speak about or bring into relationship with others. Some may edge towards intimacy through bringing 'offerings' to therapy: artwork; poetry. Henry brought an orchid grown at home, a beautiful flower nurtured in a sensitive environment, representing his Child of Self.

I end this essay with a reminder that the psychospiritual context of psychosynthesis therapy offers light at the end of the tunnel. True alignment with Self enables the individual to feel safe as she brings her qualities into the world. Although the work of facilitating disidentification can only begin when the 'I' has been safely embodied, paradoxically, working with disidentification later in therapy can help anchor the 'I' so that it does not become overwhelmed by energies from the unconscious, the superconscious or Self. The perceived experience of separation from spirit at the point of incarnation can only be resolved psychospiritually: the Sacred Wound cannot be 'repaired' through therapy but is transformed as alignment brings together heart and mind. The open heart 'sees through' into the depths of soul while the mind makes sense of and integrates what it encounters there before turning to contemplate spirit.

Once the realm of the imagination becomes as real to the lost child as the world of matter to which she is now willing to return, and vice versa, Self can be expressed through the language of the symbolic imagination. A stream of night and day dreams, images, symbols, stories and archetypes may mark the unfolding of psychological process under the direction of Self. At a time of intense grief, Lucy's long-dead grandmother came to her in a dream, accompanied by a feeling of euphoria, to tell Lucy *All is well. The purpose of your life is to live it to the full and enjoy.* At this stage of therapy, wise mentors appear in meditations bringing variations of the message that God dwells in the world, and Heaven on Earth. The individual comes to realise she really does walk between two worlds. Her rich Neverland of internal objects can at last be encouraged to work in service of the greater whole.

References

Kundera, M, *The Unbelievable Lightness of Being*, Faber and Faber, 1989

Odier, D, *Tantric Quest: An Encounter with Absolute Love*, Inner Traditions, 1997

Grof, C and Grof, S, *The Stormy Search for the Self*, Jeremy Tarcher Inc., 1990

Evans, J, 'The Triphasic Model of Psychospiritual Unfoldment', *Institute of Psychosynthesis*, 2008

Guntrip, H, *Schizoid Phenomena, Object Relations and the Self*, Hogarth Press, 1986

Winnicott, DW, *The Maturational Processes and the Facilitating Environment*, Hogarth Press, 1965

Jung, CG, 'The Collected Works of CG Jung', *Psychology Types*, Vol 6, Routledge and Kegan Paul, 1971, 2nd ed.

Johnson, S, *Character Styles*, WW Norton, 1994

Kelley-Lainé, K, Peter Pan, *The Story of Lost Childhood*, Element Books, 1997

Psychosynthesis

Risks, Opportunities and Ethical Issues for Psychospiritual Practitioners in a Changing Clinical Context

Julie O'Brien

Context

State registration of psychotherapists and increased regulation of training and practice by the main counselling association in Aotearoa New Zealand have led me to consider how to assist external bodies in understanding the importance and value of psychospiritual practice. I propose three things would support that goal: contributing to cross-modality awareness of the importance of attending to spirituality in counselling and therapy; describing what we do and how we do it in a way that is more easily understood outside psychosynthesis; and providing reassurance of client safety through deepening the discussion about ethical issues related to psychospiritual practice. This essay contributes to these three matters. Although the UK and most other countries in the world have 'voluntary registration' (Tudor, 2013, p. 50), these issues are also relevant in that context.

Spirituality in Counselling and Therapy Practice

Paradoxically, some practitioners in other modalities are identifying the need for increased awareness of spiritual issues in clinical work (see for example Bray, Thorne, West). This has been attributed to people's "lost confidence in organised religion's ability to answer all their questions" (Culbertson, 2013, p. 8), and means practitioners need "to be open to conversations about spirituality, and aware of the major do's and don'ts when the topic is raised in our professional relationships" (*ibid*). Culbertson goes further to state that the practitioner "may be functioning as the most influential spiritual guide" (*ibid*) that a client has.

Despite this, a recent review of spirituality in counsellor education in Aotearoa New Zealand noted the term 'spirituality' was rarely used in counselling training marketing, and there were few articles on this topic in the main counselling association's journal (Bray, 2011, p. 91). From my own observation, this is true also of psychotherapy journals in New Zealand and Australia. Bray concludes, "counselling in Aotearoa New Zealand has reached an evolutionary point where it can no longer ignore international debate about the inclusion and relevance of spiritual issues in counselling" (2011, p. 92).

However, it seems that even if there is 'debate' in other countries in practice, clients and practitioners are not getting their needs well met. Clients still report having medication increased when they mention spiritual conviction and hiding spiritual feelings in response to (perceived) disapproval by their therapists, while practitioners search in vain for supervision of their clinical work on spiritual issues (Thorne, 2011, p xvii). Thorne asserts, "there is continuing evidence, in short, that there remains deeply entrenched in the therapeutic profession a suspicion of and even hostility towards both clients and practitioners for whom spiritual reality constitutes their primary source of meaning and motivational energy" (2011, p xviii).

One of the problems facing those who recognise the importance of attending to spirituality in clinical work is the lack of a coherent theoretical framework. For example, West recommends Wilbur's 10-stage model of spiritual development as the 'best fit' for him, but notes the model's absolutist metaphysics as well as its lack of information about the spiritual tasks – and therefore the therapeutic work. This leaves him with only his personal experience to guide him, "knowing what is true by the process of sitting with what you believe it to be in a process of mediation, contemplation and prayer" (West, 2011, p. 219). The risk of this strategy is privileging one's own meaning making, rather than, to use Ferrer's evocative metaphor, understanding spirituality as "an ocean with many shores" (2002, p. 133).

Psychosynthesis offers specialised training based on a coherent theoretical framework and substantial body of practice, resourcing practitioners with skills and expertise to bring to cross-modality dialogue, as well as to the professional development and supervision of practitioners undertaking psychospiritual work.

Psychospiritual Approach

Assagioli defined the central purpose of psychosynthesis as "to release or, let us say, help to release, the energies of the Self. Prior to this the purpose is to help integrate, to synthesise, the individual around the personal self, and then later to effect the synthesis between the personal ego and the Self" (1980, p. 65). Self is defined as the "unifying centre" (1980, p. 21) and "luminous source" of our being (1980, p. 20). The purpose of accessing the energies of the Self is to transform self-centredness into altruistic expression in the world through service, as expressed in the phrase 'I will to will Thy will'.

Assagioli's definition indicates the developmental and ideally sequential process from attending to personal psychological issues (self-actualisation) prior to spiritual work (Self-realisation) – for those clients who wish to access this level of their experience. The exception to this is when a 'peak experience' or spiritual opening spontaneously occurs.

Psychosynthesis emerged out of Assagioli's psychoanalytic training – extending Freud's interest in 'the basement' of a person, to 'the whole building'. "We try to build an elevator which will allow a person access to every level of his personality. After all a building with only a basement is very limited. We want to open up the terrace where you can sunbathe or look at the stars" (Keen, 1976, p. 203).

Therefore, and in the spirit of 'synthesis' (i.e. placing together) this first stage of integration of the self draws on contemporary developmental models, attachment theory, trauma theory and so on, in addition to psychosynthesis, depending on the needs of the client. We attend to the client's process as well as the content of what they are saying, and also the transferential dynamics of the relationship. Psychosynthesis is therefore relationally and phenomenologically based, rather than reliant on a set of techniques to be followed in a pre-determined order.

Psychosynthesis theory differentiates and includes sensate experience, emotions and thoughts as the contents and processes of the psyche at three levels of consciousness. This includes the painful, pathological, instinctual and past experiences of the basic unconscious, the ordinary everyday conscious and readily accessible unconscious material of the middle ground, and the joy, peace and compassion of superconscious experience. Our individual experience is contextualised within the same three levels of the collective consciousness/unconscious, as well as a "socio-cultural context that extends all the way to the Universe" (Hubbard and Palmer, 2013, p. 39).

Crucially, in terms of understanding spirituality, Assagioli differentiated superconscious experiences from the spiritual Self (1980, p. 198), the point at which the individual meets the universal, even though superconscious contents and processes at the most heightened levels of awareness are not dissimilar to the characteristics of the. "The Self, on the other hand, is stable, unmoving, unchanging" (1991, p. 29), and is "enduring, immortal essence" (1991, p. 31). In the experience of Self there is "a forgetfulness of all contents of consciousness, of all which forms the personality" (1980, p. 202). Through Self, therefore, we access dimensions beyond the dynamic contents and processes of our own being.

Assagioli's differentiation accords with contemporary post-modern spirituality theory. For example, Ferrer asserts that spiritual phenomena are not merely "individual inner experiences, but...participatory events that can emerge in the locus of an individual, a relationship, a collective identity, or a place" (2002, p. 3). And Rovers and Kocum state "spirituality is better understood as a multidimensional space within which every person may be located. As such spirituality has many domains, dimensions, and definitions. Spirituality can be conceived of as the driving force which gives meaning, stability and purpose to life through relatedness to dimensions that transcend the self" (2010, p. 3).

Psychosynthesis places will as the central function and expression of the self. It has "a directive and regulatory function; it balances and constructively utilises all the other activities and energies of the human being" (Assagioli, 1973, p. 100). Through developing experiential awareness of our will, we increasingly learn how to access and direct it to express our unique contribution to the world, and align with what has purpose, meaning and value to us.

Understanding will in this way means, in terms of spirituality, that accessing higher states of consciousness and the Self through 'peak experiences' is not the ultimate purpose of spiritual practice: "The mystical experience, while having positive value is not an end in itself and is a partial experience of the spiritual life" (Assagioli, 1980, p. 207). The value of spiritual experience "has more to do with its emancipatory power for self, relationships and world (i.e. its capability to free individuals, communities, and societies from egocentric understandings of reality and associated ways of life)" (Ferrer, 2002, p. 3).

Psychosynthesis provides theoretical maps and models of consciousness and will, which guide clinical work. A key strategy of this work is to increase space and differentiation in the psyche through working with the processes of identifying and disidentifying. This requires directing will to bring awareness to moment by moment experience at the levels of body, feelings and mind, before inviting the experience of 'more than'. Hubbard notes that, "crucially, by virtue of the invitation to experience being 'more than', this is done with an invocation of space in psyche" (2013, p. 56).

By engaging with our experience of *being* in this moment, we increase our capacity to be present to both the joys and suffering of our lives, and avoid striving towards *becoming* more of our potential in an ungrounded or disconnected manner. In this way, we avoid "the privileging of a transcendent spiritual dimension of unchanging ontological experience over an immanent spiritual dimension of being embodied, and therefore, evolving" (Hubbard and Palmer, 2013, p. 39).

A focus on how a client is engaging will (consciously or unconsciously) to organise their experience, and on increasing their experience of inner space, grows their ability to hold a point of tension between inner conflicts, multiple motivations, the needs of self and others, and other intra-personal and inter-personal dynamics. In this space the ability to respond rather than react develops, to make more conscious and life enhancing choices and behave in more serving ways.

This process is both differentiating and inclusive of all aspects of experience, and therefore coheres the personality into a more unified and harmoniously functioning whole, and generates functioning as a spacious, disidentified personal centre of identity – a dynamic process that gradually becomes more sustained. At this level of psychological functioning it becomes easier to align with and open to the experience of Self, and also to integrate spiritual experiences and insights into the personality so they can be meaningfully expressed in altruistic and ethical behaviour in the world.

Considering the term psychospiritual as an adjective rather than a noun opens up a way of thinking about the different dimensions of what it is to be human, and therefore the relationship between them, i.e. the evolutionary imperative towards the expression of Self, and the psychological defences against that unfolding. This differentiation is a clinical one, as its dualism doesn't reflect the reality that Self permeates all aspects of self, and that our physical, emotional and mental experience "can be ontologically considered as dynamically cohered Spirit-as-form" (Palmer, 2012, p. 54). However, it reflects how most of us experience ourselves in ordinary waking consciousness – as distinct, but separate. When we contact Self, we know we are distinct yet not separate.

Acknowledging the interactive processes of our psychology and spirituality means psychosynthesis offers ways of understanding and working with the psychospiritual dynamics of repressing the sublime and spiritual bypassing. We have insight into the processes of spiritual awakening, in particular Assagioli's four stages of that process (1980, pp. 40-59). Psychospiritual psychology also offers us a way to understand the challenges for those on a spiritual path, such as spiritual narcissism, spiritual materialism and crises of duality, and how to differentiate spiritual emergence/awakening from spiritual crisis/emergency, and also from psychosis. Psychosynthesis practitioners, rather than pathologising a temporary reduction in functioning that can occur as a result of spiritual experience, understand the possibility of a regression in service of transcendence. By including spirituality, psychosynthesis also brings an additional dimension to understanding depression, loss of meaning and other existential issues.

Ethical Issues

Knowing the Ethical Limits of Psychospiritual Practice

Even if some practitioners are spiritual guides in other contexts, Assagioli made it clear that psychosynthesis leads to the 'door to the Mystery', and not beyond. In other words, our role is to be "an ally in spiritual exploration, rather than a spiritual teacher" (Vega, 2005, p. 64). We each need ways of ensuring we are not seduced into crossing that threshold in our clinical work, especially if we have a client who is interested in the same spiritual tradition as our own, or who wants to explore their spirituality and has no one else to guide them.

Having our Own Spiritual Practice

Can we be allies for someone else's spiritual exploration if we haven't done our own? West, while recommending therapists' "personal exposure to a variety of spiritual teaching and practices" (2011, p. 218), rejects the necessity for a personal spiritual practice (p. 219). I disagree, as I find it hard to imagine how to be an ally without having a lived experience of both the rewards and challenges of spiritual life. A spiritual path sustains us to live an ethical and responsible life personally and professionally. It helps us open to and be held by divine guidance/wisdom in our clinical work, including managing the transferential dynamics of psychospiritual work e.g. being pulled into being the guru.

So, what constitutes a spiritual path and practice? If we accept that spirituality's purpose is transformative in order to move away from egoic concerns to a more altruistic orientation, it is not merely about using practices to access a good feeling (peace/joy), nor about feeling good (virtuous), confusions not uncommonly encountered in training and clinical practice. Ferrer (2002, p. 24) notes that traditionally spiritual paths have involved a combination of individual practices (such as meditation), as well as communal life, ethical commitments, relationships with teachers, and study of scriptures. Self-created spiritual paths that are divorced from any ethical context and not grounded in some kind of lineage and community risk reinforcing narcissistic tendencies rather than activating spiritual transformation. So, the issue for each of us is how we ensure we really are practising spiritually, rather than just making ourselves feel better.

Knowing Our History, Assumptions and Defences Around Spirituality

Being able to articulate our historic and current spiritual beliefs, path and practices, and being aware of the assumptions inherent in them, helps us to disidentify from them, so that conversations in the room focus on the client's phenomenological experience and meaning making. Practitioners "who know themselves and value their own spiritual journeys are more aware of how they might influence their clients, and are more able to invite them to name these fundamental spiritual concerns safely" (Bray, 2011, p. 80). This includes knowing our own shadow and defences in relation to spirituality. Writing a spiritual biography can be a useful tool. We are just as susceptible to common psychospiritual issues as our clients, such as repressing the sublime, spiritual narcissism and spiritual bypassing. This means it is helpful to have someone who reflects us in a way that ensures we don't go blind to our own tendencies in relation to spirituality.

Having a Conceptual Framework for Understanding Other Spiritual Traditions

Another support for our work is being able to make meaning about spirituality that does not privilege the practices and beliefs of our own tradition, but maintains the 'metaphysical neutrality' Assagioli endeavoured to bring to psychosynthesis. Ferrer addressed this with his contention that "no pregiven ultimate reality exists, and that different spiritual ultimates can be enacted through intentional or spontaneous creative participation in an indeterminate spiritual power or Mystery" (2002, p. 151).

Some knowledge of other traditions is also useful, while also bringing an attitude of 'informed not knowing' to any client's process. This means disidentifying in the mental field in order to hear beliefs contrary or antagonistic to our own, and also emotionally, as faith has an emotional aspect to it. Developing both a generic framework for understanding spirituality and some wider understanding of other paths may involve reading and dialogue outside our own traditions.

Avoiding Any Tendency to Spiritualise All Experience

If our tendency is to be drawn to the spiritual work, we need to ensure our clinical practice is well grounded in the personality cohering stage of personal psychosynthesis. This includes staying current to developments in counselling and psychotherapy in general. Palmer suggests, "it is not unreasonable to assume an effective psychosynthesis practitioner should have a general knowledge of core concepts of psychodynamic personality theory, and be aware of current theoretical developments in object relations, intersubjective psychology, trauma theory, attachment theory, and neuroscience" (2012, p. 19).

Competence in Working with Spiritual Issues

Although psychosynthesis training prepares practitioners to work with psychospiritual issues, individuals have a range of confidence with these, and we each need to be clear about the limits of our competence. If we use the name psychosynthesis in our marketing, then we are implying we are psychospiritual practitioners. This means being able to work with spiritual issues as the need arises, such as spiritual crises or kundalini experiences. If we don't feel competent to, it's important to know when to refer on. The American Counselling Association, for example, has adopted the following competencies: knowledge of spiritual phenomena, awareness of one's own spiritual perspective, understanding of client's spiritual perspectives, and spiritually related interventions and strategies (cited by Bray, 2011, p. 78).

Care With What We Promise

The final issue is what we promise, either directly to clients or in our marketing. Just as we wouldn't promise to cure depression, we can't claim to bring about someone's spiritual awakening or enlightenment. The balance here is to market ourselves in ways that indicates our ability to work with spirituality without implying specific outcomes.

Conclusion

As the context in which we practice changes there are risks and opportunities for psychospiritual practitioners. Key to ensuring that the validity and importance of psychospiritual work is understood by those bodies able to influence its practice is our contribution to cross-modality dialogue, our ability to articulate well what we do and how we do it, and clarity of understanding and practice around the ethical issues inherent in psychospiritual work. In this essay, I've drawn on my own training, clinical, teaching and spiritual practice to make a contribution to those ends.

References

Assagioli, R, *Psychosynthesis: A Manual of Principles and Techniques*, Turnstone Books, 1980

Assagioli, R, *The Act of Will*, Penguin, 1973

Assagioli, R, *Transpersonal Development: The Dimension Beyond Psychosynthesis*, Thorsons, 1991

Bray, P, 'Naming Spirituality in Counselling Education: A Modest Proposal', *New Zealand Journal of Counselling: Special Issue on Counsellor Education in Aotearoa New Zealand*, New Zealand Association of Counsellors, 2011

Culbertson, P, 'Working with Spiritual Difference, or "you believe WHAT?"', *New Zealand Journal of Counselling*, 2013, Vol 2

Ferrer, J, *Revisioning Transpersonal Theory: A Participatory Vision of Human Spirituality*, State University of New York Press, 2002

Keen, S, 'The Synthetic Vision: A Conversation with Roberto Assagioli' in *Voices and Visions*, Harper and Row, 1976

Hubbard, P, 'Shaping a Psychospiritual Participatory Paradigm', *Essays on the Theory and Practice of a Psychospiritual Psychology*, Simpson, S, Evans, J, and Evans, R, (eds.) Volume 1, Institute of Psychosynthesis, 2013

Palmer, H, 'Psychosynthesis in the South Pacific: Ontological and Epistemological Considerations in the Context of Aotearoa New Zealand' in *Essays on the Theory and Practice of a Psychospiritual Psychology*, Simpson, S, Evans, J, and Evans, R, (eds.) Volume 1, Institute of Psychosynthesis, 2013

Palmer, H, *Psychosynthesis in the South Pacific: Ontological and Epistemological Considerations in the Context of Aotearoa New Zealand*, Institute of Psychosynthesis, 2012, Psychosynthesis Monograph 10

Rovers, M, and Kocum, L, 'Development of a holistic model of spirituality', *Journal of Spirituality in Mental Health*, 2010, Vol 12, pp. 2-24

Thorne, B, 'Foreword' in *Exploring Therapy, Spirituality and Healing*, West, W, (ed.), Palgrave Macmillan, 2011,

Tudor, K 'Be Careful What You Wish For', *New Zealand Journal of Counselling*, Vol 2, 2013

Vega, S, 'Breathing Into Fear: Psychospiritual Approaches for Treating Anxiety', *The Psychospiritual Clinician's Handbook: Alternative Methods for Understanding and Treating Mental Disorders*, Mijares, S, and Khalsa, GS, (eds.), The Haworth Reference Press, 2005

West, W, 'Practice Around Therapy, Spirituality and Healing' in *Exploring Therapy, Spirituality and Healing*, West, W (ed.), Palgrave Macmillan, 2011

Psychosynthesis: a Clinician's Notebook

Alignment and Healing Through the Self

Jay Ramsay

Alignment with the Self is more and more important at this time of uncertainty and change. Assagioli saw clearly that disidentification – the cornerstone exercise and practice of psychosynthesis – is the key to our psychological freedom from the drives of both our ego and our subpersonalities. Implied in his awareness (and esoteric background, of course) is the connection between Self and 'spirit' within the expansion that Self is. We are connecting with the spiritual world when we connect, when we align, with Self. My own belief is that it is time this connection was made more overt, and perhaps (in one sense) more de-mystified and less taboo as well. We should be able to talk more freely about it. And not only this: but seeing that *the Self is itself a healer* – the Self is a portal into which higher energies can and do regularly flow, and (as we say) 'download'. This also requires us to take energy more seriously as part of the therapeutic process – the invisible component, the X factor that is essential. How does the healing we experience with our clients really take place? What makes psychosynthesis a Psychotherapy of Love as Firman and Gila have asserted? What are we thinking? And how much is that healing restricted according to our own limited or overly-concretized view?

This is what I want to start exploring in this essay.

Assagioli, as often, put it in a nutshell: "What has to be achieved is to expand the personal consciousness into that of the Self". This has been a kind of mantra for my private practice over some years now, also because (in a phrase) it describes the journey of healing which is synthesis. Of course we also have to identify with the personal consciousness before we can disidentify from it, because – as he also noted in many places – there are dangers of distortion and misinterpretation on the way. But this awareness of *expansion* is basic, and it is what can get so easily lost in or work if we don't actively remember it and help our clients to practise it. For me, the beginning of a session always begins with a body/feelings/mind meditation to help facilitate not only 'self-remembering' deeper than our usual mental identifications (with our preoccupying thoughts), but also an expansion into the Self that is always with us – and that is the piece I add on. Its other practical and more personified name is 'the witness', so I will refer to it as that: 'the witnessing part of you', especially if clients are uncomfortable with notions of Higher Self, which is often the case where there is, by definition, are repression of the sublime. As Assagioli says in his important and late essay 'Transpersonal Inspiration': "Furthermore, the mind is reluctant to admit the existence of realities and values not consistent with the known rational world; *it confuses what is super-rational with what is irrational or anti-rational* [my italics]" (1973, p. 59).

The confusion of these elements is part of what goes against an understanding of the Self in the first place, and remains part of the sceptical and cynical world view still advocated in our time. In our terms it is a 'collapse of levels', but this is of course exactly what we are going to encounter in some of our clients who are not only seeking our help but who unconsciously long for a connection with the very thing they denigrate.

Dr Eben Alexander, one time atheist-neurologist, in his stunning book *Proof of Heaven* which documents his extensive NDE, furthers the case: "What I discovered out beyond is the indescribable complexity and immensity of the universe, and that *consciousness* is the basis of all that exists. I was so totally connected to it that there was often no real differentiation between 'me' and the world I was moving through" (2012).

Alexander witnesses the Self not just as an abstract concept, and certainly not merely as an archetype, but as a quantum reality. It is important that we know that what we are talking about here is real. In fact, it is the realest thing there is. And of course it has enormous consequences for how we think of our identity and the identity of the person we are sitting with…because it is real for all of us. The only distinction is how aware we are of that.

We are surrounded by something not only vaster and more loving than ourselves, but a source of love and healing that can be drawn on at any time because its energy is universal as well as local. Like the Egyptian hieroglyph for the sun – a dot surrounded by a circle – finite manifestation is surrounded by infinite source. This is not only 'proof' of the Egg Diagram, it is something more. For any practising spiritual healer, this is fundamental; and as such non-negotiable. It would be like questioning the air you breathe.

Assagioli's concern was how this superconscious reality can enter ordinary reality, and it must be and remain ours as well.

Alignment is the first aspect, which also involves an upward movement of energy through the chakras as well as a settling of physical energy within relative stillness. We literally ascend from body self to 'I' towards Self. We also return (at the end of the opening meditation I described) to the presence of mind, feelings and body. *Who* is present when we are present rather than distracted, disassociated, avoidant? Self is.

• • •

A clinical example is my work with E over a four year period during which she experienced both spiritual emergence and healing that might be more accurately be described as a recovery of the Self, as I believe she would now see it.

Her background involved an experience of having M.E. as a child of 7 in which her reality was not confirmed. She was surrounded by doctors trying to fix her rather than empathising with her: an all too common story. Later this re-surfaced in her already compromised energy (and sense of self) reaching a crisis point that resulted in Prozac, which pretty much zombified her. She came to me in recovery from this medicated state, ready to thaw out.

I will quote her in her own words since she is the best author of her own script. To begin with her experience through our therapy was of being 'broken down and reformed'. What was breaking down was her numbed state, and her identification with her limited survival personality as her authentic self started to 'grow through'. And her initial experience of this was great fear: authentic self exposed, like a snail without its shell. She says, "I was aware that my behaviours were disrupted and strange. I knew this seemed contradictory. There were pieces of it, and me. Now it feels like they are becoming whole".

And she adds "Whole me was there all along but not consciously..." For 'whole me' we can read I and Self.

Her journey was very much to do with naming splits and subpersonalities which illuminated a condition of inner division with its accompanying loss of energy. (It is always exhausting to be divided against oneself). This was her journey towards 'I'. As she says: "I wasn't relating to them ('the pieces' i.e. subpersonalities) in context". In fact at that stage she had no context. She was multiple in terms of her internal world, and under other circumstances could have become quite fragmented. "All those views (of the subpersonalities) were true if partial perceptions." Her phrasing is elegant and precise, also as a summary of subpersonalities themselves and their function within us.

In the first stage, she states, "Consciousness was flipping all over. Now the identified parts have joined up". And: "The whole forms as the parts join up".

Most significantly, then: "I'm not pulled around so I can remain in the 'I'". This of course was the replacing of her survival personality by her authentic self, appropriately supported and nurtured. It didn't happen overnight.

Later, she reflects: "Strange, but there was always a sense of safety in the background – in general that is! Quite subtle".

This is clearly much more than the therapist (me) as an external unifying centre, although of course that was significant. This is *her own* experience of Self emerging. She also says very poignantly: "I couldn't have coped if I thought it (the fragmentation) was true".

Increasingly what emerged in her though her authentic self was a sense of *presence* as well as a capacity to disidentify in a way that was natural to her intelligence as well as suggested by me. That became more and more obvious as she also recovered her capacity for intuition as well as her own mystical experiences, often in Nature – as well as one which very powerfully involved the death of a previous partner: a major experience of expansion and consciousness for her. It was as if her own experiences of and within Self *were returning as Self to her*; and of course this time her reality was being confirmed.

At the same time, she understood her social isolation. "I couldn't really relate to people. I had nothing to relate *from*". And, as compellingly: "I thought spirit was fluffy…now I see it wasn't that at all!"

Reading between the lines here, you can see what was moving for and within her; and through her own account. This resulted not just in a re-emergence of herself but in taking a number of major life decisions (including her own training) which would have previously been almost unthinkable. Self reveals itself here both vertically in terms of alignment and connection—and also horizontally in terms of action. These two dimensions of Self are very useful to bear in mind. Without 'claiming' Self—which is what the ego does—we have a connection and a presence that also allows us to perform deeds of courage as well as devotion; even, we might say 'radical action'. This has been true in her on-going story. It is also overt, for example, in the life of Nelson Mandela in his own profound transition into peacemaker: the Self in action that touches the heart through and through.

• • •

As Roger Evans once said: "If we hold the context for Self, then it can be in the room". What separates us from holding this context for ourselves? Both our mental and our emotional states and our identification with them. Quite some time ago the philosopher Søren Kierkegaard named despair as a "disrelationship to the Self" which, as a result of our identification with it, prevents us from taking a leap of faith. He also says something important for us to remember, which is that it takes *strength* to connect with Self: identification with weakness (being the victim) and self-pity work in the opposite direction. We would say it takes will, and it does. To align with Self is a choice; it may be almost a ritual activity.

Disidentification is key here, and Anne-Marie Diepveen's testimony to this is a lovely witnessing. As she says: "To me, disidentification is the key to the next level of Consciousness, the way to peace, freedom and joy. The way to save the world!" (Simpson and Evans, 2013, p. 305).

She's right. And Alain Forget, the French spiritual teacher who bases his whole work on disidentification has some very interesting things to say about it as both a psychological and a spiritual practice – something he is bringing to the business community, where it is much-needed. We are not only separated from alignment to Self as a result of our various identifications, we are also separated from our bodies, and as a result from a healing flow of energy as well. As he notes: "You will also notice the following phenomenon: when not immersed in your thoughts, your attention shifts instantaneously into an increased sensitivity towards your body. Take this opportunity to concentrate on your breathing" (2012, p. 106).

The preparation to give healing involves exactly the same thing: aligning with Self (higher vibration) and at the same time becoming acutely physically aware of subtle energy – the healing energy as it begins to arrive in my hands, as well as my awareness of what is happening in the energetic field with my client. The sustained awareness in the therapeutic space is actually the same when we are conscious of holding this context for it. As teacher of mine once said "healing isn't just where you put your hands, it's where you put your heart". Whether we have also trained in healing as psychotherapists, or not, this kind of bi-focal vision (simultaneously of therapy ***and*** healing) I think is essential not only in terms of Self but where psychotherapy itself is going, and – as Annemarie suggests – its next level of Consciousness.

Psychosynthesis, both as a philosophy as well as a psychology (because it is both) is a perfect paradigm for this.

Our positioning as practitioners is vital here. We hold a context for Self, for healing: we consciously work on all levels within the awareness of the wholeness of our clients; we work intuitively within an intelligence that is also guided from a higher level; and above all we work with Love, and we model that through unconditional love. Love is the best healer. Its absence in the therapy room, while it might also mirror a lack of love and self-love in the client, is always an absence of necessary relationship – and in the end, necessary equality between therapist and client. Love is no friend of inequality. This is also how Love comes into the room – not romantic love, although that transference may need to be part of it, *but the Love that is the Self when it connects through the heart.* Soul to soul. Being to being.

Hester Seddon's essay on a psychospiritual approach to healing work (Simpson and Evans, 2013, p. 243) is also very significant here: I'm on the same page with her. All I would add is that we need to be careful as therapists that we don't make our clients feel that we have something they haven't got. The point is, we all have it (to whatever acknowledged degree); and without that, the real magic of what can take place in the room would never happen. It is always an interactive, co-creative field. Self and Self combine.

• • •

This dismantling or deconstructing and rebuilding, characterised by our understanding of the therapeutic process as being both regression and emergence – simultaneous arrows pointing forwards and back – is what allows Self to come into the work as well as the room.

P, another client who has suffered from long term personal anxiety and social anxiety disorder, slowly gained the ground of Self within himself in naming his wounded inner child and bullied teenager; in claiming the choice to be himself freed from his rigid Catholic upbringing (where as the eldest child it was also hardest to be authentic) as well as memories of sexual abuse as the smallest member of his rugby team. Instinctively, and despite family ambition and expectation, he chose a job working as a gardener to bring him closer to Nature and his own nature; meanwhile haunted by the memories of relationship failure partly as a result of the 1970's culture where everything was available too quickly and too soon on a drunken plate. He was never (despite his good looks) a Lothario anyway. His literally 'not knowing who I really am or was' in all this ego and superego confusion has been addressed through alignment: watching his sense of self grow in recognizing his defaults and defences has taken place beside his ability to penetrate his own anxiety, also from a place of increased embodiment and validated sensitivity.

I have watched him slowly becoming himself, and, without any religious or overt spiritual conviction, experience Self as the change he has experienced: the foundation for expanding his social contact and approaching relationships with women in a new way. I still invite him to contact the witnessing part of him 'from one step back within that feeling of expansion'.

Addiction is perhaps the biggest challenge for this work and its context, especially given the 'addictive' aspect we all have that keeps us identified with parts of ourselves at the expense of the whole. The struggle between Self and Addict is the central drama of addiction (as Craig Nakken (1988) has observed), where the negative alignment with the object or substance of the addiction is the Calf of Gold (Moses is the Self on the mountain). The choice between Self and Addict is ultimately a matter of faith (in Self): it cannot be made by the ego alone. The choice of Self, and then its betrayal (in relapse) cries out for Self to become more real, more tangible...a cry the Addict will never hear or believe in until its wreckage, its lack of expansion as well as loving relationship, becomes inescapable. We just think we can get away with it. As therapists, we model Self, as well as authentic human response and love, as a mirror to addictive distortion (someone stoned in your therapy room), within the understanding that the soul in everyone has its own journey and timing. We can incite it, encourage it, catalyse it, but we can't control it. But this holding of another being *is exactly what the Self does for us* (every day of our lives); which is useful to remember when the work is tough.

Addictions always need replacing. The triumph of Self can manifest in numerous ways through a healing that allows the gifts and qualities in our client, held within its dimension, to take its place.

There is one other area of distortion here that feels important to name, which is where ego hijacks the Self and (as I've already mentioned) claims it for its own. The result is always inflation, grandiosity – and even, in extreme cases, psychosis which is characterized by an inability to listen or receive the reality of another person or their point of view. This is really a kind of Anti-Self that we find in the use of higher energies for personal power, both in history (Hitler is the obvious example with his horrific pseudo-spirituality—the 'Self' apparently speaking to a nation) and sadly still in the present where so much is necessarily being cleared and made transparent in the collective. I was viciously attacked last year by a fundamentalist Evangelical, accused of 'worshipping other gods' and being 'full of Satan' – my libertarian and radical view of Christianity, also in my poetry, was far too threatening. The person in question had claimed to have an Near Death Experience (as a result of a genuine life-threatening illness), which made him highly persuasive until I realized what was actually going on. His emotional terrorism was of course the absolute antithesis of psychotherapy (which he despised: Jesus did it for free) as well as empathy: his alignment to the Holy Spirit took place in the complete absence of any self-reflective awareness as well as his impact on a personal and psychic level. He had been 'born again', he argued, so he had no shadow. As Shakespeare (2005) put it in *Julius Ceasar*: "Such men are dangerous". There was a very strange moment when I realized that people claiming to be of the Light and people proud of their allegiance to the Dark can merge and become the same thing…it was the Self, for me, that was witnessing this – as well as the loving witness of several spiritual friends.

It is clear that in cases like these any therapeutic work (once some aspect of deflation has taken place, that is) has to be with a client's split-off humanness: the alignment to Self in this sense is 'reversed', pointing inwards and down, until there is a readiness to recognize what we serve, in all humility. I imagine Jesus washing his feet.

References

Assagioli, R, 'Transpersonal Development' (new translation), *Smiling Wisdom*, 2007

Alexander, Dr E, *Proof of Heaven – A Neurosurgeon's Journey into the Afterlife*, Piatkus, 2012

Forget, A, *How to Get Out of This World Alive*, 2012. Available from www.alainforget.com

Nakken, C, *The Addictive Personality*, Hazelden, 1988

Ramsay, J, Anamnesis – The Remembering of Soul. Available from www.jayramsay.co.uk

Shakespeare, W, Julius Caesar, Penguin Books, 2005

Simpson, S and Evans, R (eds.) *Essays in the Theory and Practice of a Psychospiritual Psychology*, Vol 1, Institute of Psychosynthesis, 2013

Sound in the Therapy Room

Jess Curtis

Introduction

How far do we pay attention to the value of sound? As practising psychotherapists we take care in making the therapy space look, and maybe smell, welcoming, perhaps light a candle – but to what extent do we consider the soundscape?

This discourse sets out to explore the lack of aural awareness in therapeutic practice; to look at how this can be recognized and redressed; how increasing attention to the aural aspect of our work can expand and deepen the process and practice of therapy through ways of working with vocal sound, and understanding ways in which the unconscious can become conscious through raising awareness of the effects of sound on body, feelings, and soul.

Context

The customary mode of the therapeutic exchange is verbal, and so aligns itself with an oral culture which has been in existence since man acquired language. Historically, there have been three quantum leaps in communications, each of them causing strong reaction to change; from orality to writing, from writing to printing and from printing to electronics. Over centuries, we have moved from a predominantly oral culture to a visual one; and it could be that we are now on the verge of seeing the spoken word eclipsed by the cyber world. Instead of living human contact, people can turn to chat rooms, where no sound exists; children in isolation from each other can play in virtual worlds, where there may be sound effects, but, as yet, no spoken words. Consequently, there are concerns that social bonding, which used to be generated by communication between members of the family and community, is being replaced by technology with the result that the ability to communicate verbally is severely affected. The loss of this ability has repercussions for the 'talking therapies' as now we are beginning to pick up on these difficulties created by lack of development of oral language and communication skills.

We live in a world of increasingly loud unwanted sound. We often have to defend ourselves against continuous, intrusive noise, ranging from traffic to Muzac. One effect can be that we defend ourselves by blotting out these sounds – to become deaf to them. Daniel Barenboim in his 2002 Reith lecture calls hearing the 'neglected sense' because of the emphasis our culture places on the visual. And at the same time, the increasing virtual world is one in which the human voice is heard less and less; the consequence is that while we hear we may tend not to listen.

Mind

Psychotherapies have inherited from the Jungian and Psychosynthesis tradition a vast repertoire of the visual in terms of symbol, image and dream, guided meditations and drawing; this has resulted in an imbalance between the visual and the aural. This is reflected in the literature – by the fact that while we may 'tune in' to and 'resonate' with clients, most of the metaphors we use are visual, and may not be taking into account that a client may be more aurally than visually aware and receptive.

There are many books about music in therapy, but almost no references to sound or voice in the text or indices in books on psychotherapy and counselling; this is reflected in the small number of references for this article. The one exception I have found was Nina Coltart, who, in *Slouching Towards Bethlehem* (1992 p. 123), has one reference to voice where she detects *a kind of scornfulness, in a slight change of tone in his well-modulated and unrevealing voice*; but there is no reference to voice or tone in the index, which reflects a notable lack of awareness by both editor and author towards the aural.

In the therapy room there can be many intrusive sounds over which the therapist has no control – such as passing traffic, telephones, ticking clocks and noisy water pipes which need to be made conscious and included, so that attention to inner work will not be distracted. However, exterior sounds notwithstanding, the dominant sounds in the room are the voices of therapist and client. Attentive listening can enable therapists to tune in to what a client needs to be heard. How we listen to our clients and to our inner selves depends on the importance we place on the sound of the voice in relation to the words.

Associations with a vocal tone or timbre can produce strong positive or negative reactions on behalf of both therapist and client. We all unconsciously make assumptions when we hear voices and accents, and form hypotheses based on associations from the past, some positive, some negative. It can be a useful self-supervision exercise when working with counter-transference for a therapist to register and questions reactions to a client's voice.

It can be interesting to consider how clients might be hearing us. Do we sound welcoming or bored? Discussing this point with colleagues led to us listening to and some of us re-recording our answer-phone messages.

The psychotherapist Rachel Charles considers that, from the outset it can be well worth turning the attention away from the sense of the words to tune in to the ways they are spoken: "What about the non-verbal message behind the greeting? This might be conveyed by the pitch or tone of voice, the volume or the pacing of the words. A flat monotone is often linked with depression, loudness or harshness with aggression, edginess with nervousness, breathiness with sexuality, a high pitch with excitability or childlike feelings" (2004, pp. 82-3).

Many of the sounds coming from the client are wordless and can be devalued by those who are more attached to words than their meaning. In childhood, these phatic sounds, which include the ever-present *Mms* and *Ahs*, together with laughter and crying, are echoed by the mother. Within the therapeutic mother/baby dyad, there are important, often unconscious, non-verbal clues to feelings. The Jungian analyst Mary Lynn Kittlesson describes this process as "a back-and-forth, ear-based contact, where speech is, first of all, a carrier of sound" (1996, p. 228).

We need to listen consciously for clues which signal the client's true feelings. True feelings can be unintentionally exposed; they can also be masked. To quote Jung: "Voices are treacherous; they reveal far too much. You marvel at the fantastic efforts people make to sound gay, fresh, welcoming, enterprising, jolly, benevolent, full of comradeship, and so on. And you know it is merely an attempt to cover up the real truth" (*ibid*, p. 83).

If we are taken up with meaning we risk not being present to the feelings that words often mask. A research lecturer provided the following example: when he was a participant in a Gestalt workshop, the group was involved in an exercise where they rotated in concentric circles and imparted some basic information to the person who stopped opposite them. The participant happened to find himself facing the group leader and told her his name and proceeded to give her more information about himself. To his surprise and consternation she interrupted him with the words "I *not* need soothing". This had nothing to do with the content of what he was saying but it alerted him to what he had been unconsciously transmitting.

A keen aural awareness for inflection can enable therapists to perceive the underlying meaning. The ability to dis-identify clears the way for placing the attention to listening where the client's feelings really are.

Body

Hearing in evolutionary terms was the last of the senses to be perfected; but it is the first of the senses to develop in the womb and the last to remain with the dying.

There is an important difference between hearing and listening. The brain works to make sense of what we hear – listening is how we employ hearing – how we give it meaning. Tomatis (1991, p. 150) has defined hearing as passive in relation to the active qualities of listening: *The listening function does not only affect the ear. It mobilises the entire nervous system.* Listening is what we do with our ability to hear. To paraphrase a psychosynthesis saying: *We do not hear things as they are; we hear them as we are.*

How do we experience making and receiving sound? Inayat Khan stated that there is no greater and more living resonance of sound than the human body; and that is no comparison between a voice and an instrument: "…It is not true that a person hears sound only through his ears; he hears sound through every little pore of his body. It permeates through his whole being, and according to its particular influence it either slows the rhythm or it quickens the rhythm of the blood circulation; it either wakens the nervous system or it soothes it…the movement, the glance, the touch, even the breath…do not reach so far…as the voice reaches…" (1991, p. 83).

At a time when neuroscience hardly existed it is impressive that Inayat Khan was able to make this connection between sound and the nervous system.

There are many different ways in which sound is experienced by our body which is in itself a resonating instrument. Sounds are carried by vibrations; they can heal and they can destroy. Singers can shatter a wine-glass when the glass receives vibrations of an intensity that exceeds its resistance. Japanese Samuri learn a vocal sound that can stun their opponents long enough to penetrate their guard.

Feeling

Sounds can also awaken, soothe: David in the Old Testament story calms King Saul's psychotic rages by playing the harp.

Rhythm is an intrinsic component of our being. Rhythm can also calm and soothe, relaxing tense muscles; mothers have rocked babies to sleep throughout the ages. Awareness of rhythm begins in the womb where the fetus experiences the mother's heartbeat. The rocking rhythms of lullabies are used world-wide to reassure fretful children. Repetition in itself generates rhythm. And repetition is a key feature in therapy in the form of reflecting and mirroring back, for example, awareness that a point on the spiral has come round again, because the client is repeating earlier matter. Repetition is important because, without it, learning and hence its integration can be lost. Sounds, unlike the written text, are not permanent; they fade. Once a sound has faded, it is gone and can only be remembered. So repetition has always been a strategy to retain sounds in the memory and give purpose to repeated sounds in the form of chanting. Repetition enables the sound to renew, re-form and resonate in the body.

There is a strong connection between listening to a story and the process of therapy; in both the listener can hear rhythms and cadences that express struggle, fear, pain and joy as the stories unfold. Therapists are aware of its role in the mother/baby dyad. Re-creating these conditions in the therapy room is an essential part of the initial stages of therapy.

Story-telling can share many features with therapy; Clients can find reassurance via the re-creation, recycling and repetition of being listened to, heard and mirrored – particularly those who present with failed attachment or separation issues – who struggle to locate feelings they have never expressed and the words to describe them.

Stories have existed within all cultures, from earliest times. According to Pinkola Estes, in *The Gift of Story*: "Like night dreams, stories often use symbolic language, therefore passing the ego and persona, and travelling straight to the spirit and soul who listen for the ancient and universal instructions imbedded there. Because of this process, stories can teach, correct errors, lighten the heart and the darkness, provide psychic shelter, assist transformations and heal wounds" (1993).

Asking clients born before the 1980s to share their childhood play experience we get a picture of largely unsupervised, unstructured outdoor freedom in which they learned social skills. Many of these clients have also experienced the ritual of bed-time stories – the oral telling of traditional fairy stories to young children by parents or carers, so passionately advocated by Bettelheim (1998, pp. 150-6).

Asking clients to remember their earliest sounds has often brought into the room the voice of a grandmother or older relation who has had the time to be with, connect to and listen and respond to the child – and tell them stories.

Therapists, in their role of external unifying centre, hold clients until they can accept and mother themselves. An example – a therapist whose client needed support between sessions, recorded a lullaby for her to listen to in the following week, thus providing her with an aural 'transitional object'.

Clients, over time, can integrate their therapist's voice: one client told his therapist that when he faces what was a difficult situation for him, he recalls the sound of her voice and what she might be saying to him; later on in the therapy that voice will become his own.

Working with sound in dream-work can add a rich layer of exploration, such as inviting figures in the dream to speak – and placing importance on what the voices carry in terms of volume, pitch, pace, tone and inflection. Does what clients expect to hear match with what they might actually hear? As an example, one of my clients brought in a dream in which there was a lion-figure of which she was very frightened; but when I asked her to listen quietly for what sound her lion might be making, she listened for some time, and then with a face that shone with astonishment said, 'He's purring!'.

Jung advocated not only listening to inner voices but actually 'talking back', a model which was a forerunner of Gestalt chair work and psychosynthesis Sub Personality model. Encouraging clients to liberate these voices can facilitate the process of integrating them. Listening to inner voices can be important for therapist and client, both inter- and intra-personally – the sounds of inner commentary from juxtaposed and oppositional Sub Personalities.

Working with these sub-personalities and the different vocal energies they produce provides a rich ground for revealing clients' feelings – energy changes of pitch and pace when clients move from one personality to another: the wounded child, the judgmental voice of the superego, the imperious tones of the narcissist – the varied tensions between oppositional sub-personalities. This can also be a place where clients can vocally reflect an I/Self connection.

Soul

The musician Herbert Whone (2000, p. 204) suggests that a human voice can be like a harmonic of a Fundamental Tone. A parallel with psychosynthesis is to experience Self as the fundamental tone and the 'I' as the responding harmonic. Sound becomes a conduit for spirit and spirit a conduit for Self.

As the therapy moves to the transpersonal, recognising and working with a client's authentic voice is a key part of the journey. When clients connect to this part of themselves they bring self-empowerment in the recognition of their spiritual potential. Every Psychosynthesis counsellor and therapist who has shared with me their experiences when clients have touched an authentic part of themselves, hear it very clearly:

- It impacts, comes from the heart, not head, the voice is 'straighter'
- It goes from very pinched to being deep down here
- Coming from deep down and then going straight out of the forehead
- The tone is deeper, a different shade, quieter, less brittle, coming from a different place
- It has integrity and containment
- I absolutely jump with excitement that they've found this place within them. It comes from a place of authority
- It comes from the Self with a big S

Whatever the level of vocal delivery the above statements reflect an unmistakable resonance.

Conclusion

At the turn of the last century, Rudolph Steiner, the German educationalist, predicted: "There will come a time when a diseased condition will not be described as it is today by physicians and psychologists, but will be spoken of in musical terms, as one would speak of a piano that is out of tune" (Quoted by Karpf, 2006, p. 275).

Although Steiner's prediction has not yet been fully realised, the value of sound as a healing agent is beginning to be medically acknowledged through neuroscience.

By raising consciousness of, and implementing aurality in our work, we can become more sensitive to the sound of our clients being 'out of tune' with themselves and the world. In doing this we will be restoring an imbalance between the senses; and also moving nearer to Assagioli's trust that: "...the magic of sound, scientifically applied, will contribute in ever greater measure to the relief of human suffering, to a higher development and a richer integration of the human personality" (1993, p. 260).

References

Assagioli,R, *Psychosynthesis, a Manual of Principles and Techniques*, Aquarian/ Thorsons, 1993

Bettelheim, B, *The Uses of Enchantment, the Meaning and Importance of Fairytales*, Peregrine Books, 1988

Butterton, M, *Listening to Music in Psychotherapy*, Radcliffe Publishing, 2008

Charles, R, *Intuition in Psychotherapy and Counselling*, Whurr Publishers, 2004

Cox, T, *Sonic Wonderland: A Scientific Odyssey of Sound*, Bodley Head, 2013

Goldman, J, *Healing Sounds*, Element 1992

Grosz, S, *The Examined Life*, Vintage, 2003

Karpf, A, *The Human Voice*, Bloomsbury, 2006

Khan, HI, *The Mysticism of Sound and Music*, Vol 2, Element, 1991

Kittelson, ML, *Sounding the Soul*, Daimon, 1996

Palmer, S, *Toxic Childhood: How the Modern World is Damaging our Children and What We Can Do About it*, Orion 2007

Pearce, S, *The Alchemy of Voice*, Hodder & Stoughton, 2005

Pinkola Estes, *The Gift of Story*, Rider, 1993

Rodenburg, P, *The Right to Speak*, Methuen, 1992

Tomatis, A, *The Conscious Ear*, Station Hill Press, 1991

Whone, H, 'Music – the Way Out of the Maze' in *Music: Physician for Times to Come*, Campbell, D (ed.), Quest Books, 2000

Psychosynthesis and the Addictions Recovery Process

Richard Schaub and Bonney Gulino Schaub

Psychosynthesis, because its central concepts are self-knowledge, choice, and spiritual development, can contribute to the effectiveness of a person's recovery from addiction. Alcohol, cocaine, heroin, anti-anxiety agents and painkillers are all addictive; and additionally there are addictions without alcohol or drugs, including eating disorders, gambling and sex and pornography addiction, which follow the same dynamic of obsession and compulsion. In this article we refer to alcoholism as representative of all addictions.

Alcoholism is a mental obsession that leads to a physical compulsion (Alcoholics Anonymous, 1976). The person's obsessive thoughts about alcohol activate the compulsion to consume alcohol and originate when the person discovers that alcohol relieves their anxiety and vulnerability and makes them feel relaxed. The physical compulsion can become extreme: if it were physically possible, the alcoholic person would never stop drinking. Danté's image of Cerberus in the realm of gluttony in the *Inferno* is a perfect depiction of this compulsive energy (Danté, 1984, Canto 6).

The immediate question presents itself: why does a person become obsessed with alcohol? Most people can enjoy alcohol without becoming obsessed. What makes the alcoholic different? To answer this, we need to review the theoretical models of addiction.

Models of Addiction

The authors have identified at least eleven theoretical models of addiction (Schaub, and Schaub, 1997, pp. 20-27):

The Medical Model: The person has been consuming significant amounts of alcohol over a long period of time. Deprived of it, the person's central nervous system goes into a state of physiological craving (withdrawal). To suppress the craving, the person must continue alcohol consumption.

The Genetic Disease Model: The person has a genetic, bio-chemical predisposition to alcoholism, which is activated by the use of alcohol.

The Self-Medication Model: Perhaps due to trauma, the person experiences an intolerable degree of fear in daily life. He uses alcohol to soothe his anxiety.

The Dysfunctional Family Model: The person learned from people in his family that one copes with anxiety and/or depression by consuming alcohol.

The Psychosexual Development Model: The infant did not experience adequate nurturing at the oral phase of development and becomes psychologically fixated at that stage. The adult form of the oral fixation is the consuming of alcohol.

The Ego Psychology Model: Deprived of adequate nurturing and mirroring as an infant, the person has weak ego strength and cannot tolerate the pressures of life. Alcohol relieves the pressure.

The Character Defect Model: An early model offered by the 12-Step Programme of Alcoholics Anonymous (1952, p. 6) proposed that alcoholics are morally and characteriologically 'defective' and require alcohol to pacify their 'self-centered fears'.

The Instant Gratification Model: Alcoholics have a low threshold for frustration and need instant satisfaction of their impulses. This impulsiveness is reinforced by the hurried pace and empty materialism of modern life.

The Trance Model: This is based on the pleasure principle. Once the brain has experienced the pleasure of intoxication, it stores the experience like a hypnotic suggestion and desires to repeat it.

The Transpersonal-Intoxication Model: Based on the observed connection between artists and alcoholism, this model's thesis is that the alcoholic 'thirst' is really a spiritual thirst for expanded consciousness.

The Transpersonal-Existential Model: This model accepts that the human condition is innately vulnerable and anxious; and that, alcoholicsexperience this existential anxiety more acutely.

These models are greatly simplified. Their theme, though, is clear. Essential feelings of vulnerability cause or contribute to the development of addiction. This emphasis on vulnerability is verified for the authors by thirty years of clinical experience with hundreds of people in recovery. Patients repeatedly describe that the onset of their addiction was their first discovery that alcohol took away their fears and make them feel normal. Therefore, therapeutic attention must be given to the person's vulnerability in order help him recover successfully.

Early Treatment Principles

No therapist has the power to stop an alcoholic from drinking. Other factors – the family, the person's doctor, the employer, the use of rehabilitation centres – must be involved in the initial treatment of the alcoholic. The therapist becomes significant when the actual drinking has stopped and the person has detoxified.

Once detoxified, the alcoholic is technically a person in the recovery process. But an alcoholic without alcohol is now exposed to the pain of life without his 'medicine' and will return to alcohol for relief from his vulnerability. This accounts for the many early relapses in alcohol treatment. 'Relapse' – the return to drinking – is a typical part of the early recovery process. Neither the patient nor the therapist should be disheartened by relapse. It is understandable in view of the enormous life-change the alcoholic is beginning.

Early therapy should be psychoeducational. The recovering person needs to be taught new ways of thinking and behaving. The individual therapist may be capable of accomplishing this if he sees the recovering person frequently during each week. If this is not feasible, then the therapist should be sure to have the person engage in the 12 Step program of Alcoholics Anonymous or another group psychoeducational process. The success of 12 Step Programmes is that they offer an accepting community in which the cognitions and behaviours of sobriety are repetitiously taught. For example, when the recovering person notices that he is again obsessing about alcohol, he is taught to call another person in the 12 Step Programme – a 'sponsor' – and to tell the sponsor about the impulse to drink.

If the person accepts the 12-Step guidance, he literally begins to build a new identity – a 'sober' person. He doesn't yet feel like a sober person, but he accepts that he must imitate the thinking and behaviors of a sober person in order to save his life. He thinks and feels 'as if' he is a sober person. This 'sober' identity needs to become supported and reinforced so that it can stand up to the old, established pattern of alcoholic thinking and behaving. If successful in building this identity, the person in recovery will literally hear the two sides – the sober one and the old alcoholic one – arguing in his mind.

Psychosynthetic Psychotherapy

When this new sober sub-personality is minimally established through psychoeducation and/or a 12 Step program, psychosynthetic psychotherapy can begin.

Immediately, the psychosynthetic understanding of inner energies and the cultivation of new inner self-images can be used to reinforce the new sober sub-personality. Therapeutic imagery can potentiate the person's identification with the sober sub-personality by imaginally rehearsing sober thinking and sober behaviours in the various scenes of his current life. He can also utilize imagery as a negative reinforcement – imaginally rehearsing what his life will become if he returns to alcohol: in 12 Step Programmes, they call this negative reinforcement "thinking through a drink" (Schaub and Schaub, 1997). One patient wanted help in remembering that, driving drunk, he had almost killed a little girl. *Talking about it* made him feel uncomfortable, but when he actually *imagined* images of killing her with his car, he began to sob. In his tears, he renewed his commitment to staying sober.

It is also at this stage that the study of his vulnerability should begin. Despite everything he has learned in early recovery, it will be intolerable feelings of vulnerability that will cause him to relapse, to return to alcohol.

The alcoholic numbed his emotions for many years. In early recovery, he will not know how he feels or be a good reporter of his feelings to his therapist. He will need the therapist's help in developing a basic vocabulary for his emotions. Later on in this process, Assagioli's emphasis on the power of self-observation – cultivating awareness – will become central to the naming of emotions, urges, impulses, etc., but for now the therapist must be the observer and name emotions for the newly sober person.

Fight/Flight Symptoms

To assist the therapist in discerning the patient's vulnerability, the following list, describing the typical fight/flight symptoms and patterns in the recovering alcoholic, can be helpful. As the therapist hears some of the listed fight/flight symptoms in his patient, he will be hearing the disguised forms of vulnerability. Fight or flight are, of course, the two primal instincts of any human being when he feels unsafe and vulnerable: the recovering alcoholic will display many intense symptoms of fight and/or flight. The patient will not be able to describe the subtleties of vulnerability, but he will be able to tell you that he wanted to beat up his boss (fight) or that she ate a gallon of ice cream (flight) after her boy friend argued with him.

Fight

Mental Patterns of Fight: Rigidity, obsessiveness, lack of creativity, black and white thinking, judgmentalism, intolerance, fanaticism, hyper-vigilance, arrogance, manipulativeness.

Physical Patterns of Fight: Hypertension, headaches, gastrointestinal disturbances, chronic muscle tension, rigid diets, body armoring, workaholism, forcing body to exceed limits (e.g., risk taking, extreme exercise).

Emotional Patterns of Fight: Constricted affect, rigid control of feelings, grandiosity, fake performance of feelings, denial of vulnerability, overly aggressive, rageful, domineering

Spiritual Patterns of Fight: Self-righteous, fundamentalism, dogmatism, attempts to control other people's inner lives, negation of spirituality.

Flight

Mental Patterns of Flight: Chronic refusal to decide, numbed mental processes, disconnection, dissociation, self-depreciation, victimized thinking, unthinking acceptance of others' opinions and demands, indifference, inability to focus, self-pity, self-absorption.

Physical Patterns of Flight: Low energy, compulsive TV watching, repetitive self-soothing, overeating, immobilization, avoidance, isolation, lack of self-care.

Emotional Patterns of Flight: Helplessness, hopelessness, emotional flooding, guilt and shame, unworthiness, co-dependence.

Spiritual Patterns of Flight: Magical thinking, narcissistic theology, non-directed, superficial spiritual dabbling, emptiness, lack of relatedness to a larger vision of life, lack of trust in his own experiences, lack of meaning or purpose.

When a pattern of fight and/or flight is recognised, the therapist can then investigate the incident that triggered this reaction. Predictably, the incident will reveal a vulnerable moment. The patient who wanted to beat up his boss was asked to go back into his memory and to see what triggered his impulse to fight. He saw in his memory that his fight reaction was the result of a mild criticism from the boss. The patient who ate a gallon of ice cream saw in her memory that her flight reaction was triggered the moment her boy friend's appeared bored with her. Gaining recognition of the impact of criticism or inattention moves the therapy toward the core issue of vulnerability itself, rather than staying focused on the incident with the boss or boy friend.

The Balance and Synthesis of Opposites

In psychosynthetic terms, we can view fight and flight as polarities, as two extreme and opposite reactions to vulnerability. There is nothing inherently wrong with either polarity in a specific situation. The mental pattern of arrogance (fight), for example, may be helpful when we need to assert ourselves. The mental pattern of self-depreciation (flight) may be helpful when we need to go along with a group decision. Problems develop when we habitually utilize one extreme or the other and have no capacity to consciously choose when to use them.

The goal is not to get rid of the polarities, which would be impossible anyway, but rather to use the positive aspects of their energies. Assagioli's insight into the balance and synthesis of opposites is an ideal and remarkably non-judgmental way to work with these polarities. He notes that "psychological life can be regarded... as continual effort, conscious or not, to establish equilibrium" (1975, p. 5). For example, a positive aspect of arrogance can be personal pride and a positive aspect of self-depreciation can be humility. Assagioli (*ibid*) suggests that if we could synthesize these positive aspects of arrogance and self-depreciation, i.e. if we could synthesize the energies of personal pride and humility, we would be cultivating dignity – a highly desirable quality. This psychosynthetic understanding of the refinement and transformation of inner possibilities leads the patient toward skills that will serve him again in his spiritual development. We will address this later in the article.

Emotional Development in Recovery

The therapist's focus on the patient's experiences of vulnerability will in time help the patient to recognize those vulnerable moments for himself. With this increased self-knowledge as the groundwork, the patient then needs to learn new, healthier responses to his moments of vulnerability, rather than continue in patterns of fight/flight reactivity.

The therapist should not assume that the patient will know any healthy adaptive responses; he was using alcohol all the years when others were learning how to cope with the anxieties of being alive. There is a formula: the age at which the alcoholic began heavy drinking is the age of his present emotional development. For example, if he was drinking heavily by age sixteen, your patient may be chronologically forty-two but he is emotionally a sixteen year old.

There are five important goals in this stage of the therapy. Two are concepts that should be taught and discussed until the patient can integrate them.

The first concept is 'feelings aren't facts': Borrowed from the 12 Step Programme, this establishes that, although you may feel unsafe and vulnerable in a certain situation, it does not mean that you are actually unsafe. The concept tries to modify the trigger between vulnerability and fight/flight, calming down the patient's instinctive reactions and increasing the ability to choose his responses to feeling vulnerable.

The second concept is the normalcy of shifting feelings: The normal moment-to-moment flow of changing thoughts and moods can feel too unstable to the person in recovery. He needs to understand and be reassured that the flux of change is normal and not a cause for worry. His years of alcoholism have prevented him from learning this fact of emotional life. He may, for example, report that he got very upset and didn't know what to do. The 'normal' person knows that he or she can get upset and that he or she will survive it. The recovering alcoholic interprets being upset as a danger signal and an indication that he can't live without alcohol.

The third goal of this stage of therapy is teaching stress management skills: These are the healthier responses to feeling vulnerable. In general, they will be variations on meditation and imagery, but must be pragmatic skills that the patient can do anytime, anyplace. Yoga postures will not be possible on the bus, but a simple breathing technique will work well and go unnoticed. Many of our patients like this simple phrase which they repeat silently in their mind: "_____ (their first name), let go". In the post-traumatic stress of Manhattan since September 11th many patients use this phrase as they enter the subway, cross a bridge, ride in an elevator, or see a plane in the sky. In the psychosynthetic spirit of working collaboratively, the therapist and patient can experientially try out many stress management skills and discover which ones work best.

The fourth goal of emotional development is the need for a second recovery: This is the need to recover from trauma. In the authors' experience, the majority of alcoholics have significant trauma in their early years of development. This is not typically dealt with in drug and alcohol treatment centres, but needs to be part of the psychotherapeutic view of recovery from addictions. This second recovery is of course a long-term process. It is aided by the repeated corrective experiences the patient can have with a psychosynthetic therapist who sees the 'alcoholic' as only a sub-personality in a much greater view of who the patient is.

The fifth goal is the recovery of intuition: Intuition originates in a place of deep wisdom and knowing in human nature. It is an aspect of the psychosynthetic concept of the Higher Self. By helping the patient to re-discover their intuition, he gains another tool in transcending his fight/flight reactivity and instead has a wiser level of mind available to deal with vulnerable moments.

Spiritual Development

Deriving from the 12-Step Programme's emphasis on spirituality, many alcohol treatment centres encourage some form of spiritual development as part of the recovery process. The word 'spirituality' is carefully chosen to distinguish it from religion. Spirituality is a series of expansions of identity in which the person realizes that he is participating in a larger life than his separate, anxious, self-absorbed personality. This 'larger life' may be described as God, but 12 Step Programmes are careful to say "God as you understand God" (Alcoholics Anonymous, 1952).

Psychosynthesis offers many advantages at this stage of recovery. Through Assagioli's elegant integration of psychological and spiritual insights and methods, the psychosynthetic therapist can assist the patient toward discoveries of higher consciousness without the need for any pre-formed ideas about spirituality. Assagioli saw higher consciousness as an obvious fact: "We consider that the spiritual is as basic as the material part of man" (1965, p. 193).

By discovering, through direct experience, the patient's natural spirituality, the patient can form his own spiritual understandings. He may search out many schools of spirituality, but the psychosynthetic therapist has helped the patient to have his own experiences as his guide. In psychosynthesis the primary methods for spiritual development are:

- A thorough understanding of Assagioli's map of consciousness
- The cultivation of awareness, of the 'I-space'
- The learned ability to disidentify from negative and self-defeating patterns
- The meditative use of transpersonal symbols
- The confidence that a higher, saner aspect of our nature – our Higher Self – is guiding our evolution

The authors' clinical experience shows that true spiritual development must be rooted in direct experience. Patients who have adopted a spiritual or religious perspective but have not directly experienced its truths gain no benefit from it when a crisis comes along. Spiritual development must come from lived experience.

The issue next arises: what is a spiritual experience? People can have many non-ordinary experiences which do not necessarily contribute to their spiritual development: people in recovery have experienced many altered states of consciousness via drugs, and yet none of these altered states has helped them to develop spiritually. After the examination of many Eastern and Western spiritual experiences and maps, the authors found in *The Divine Comedy* an elegant and comprehensive view of higher consciousness (Schaub and Schaub, 2003).

Danté's Pilgrim experiences two types of higher consciousness – the guiding wisdom of Beatrice, and the liberation from the personality into states of illumination. Wisdom and illumination in turn lead the Pilgrim to unitive consciousness, to enlightenment. The authors found it intriguing that all of the Pilgrim's illuminations are expansions of consciousness into the energy field. Danté utilizes many descriptions of radiance and light to describe these expansions. Although considered a Catholic poet, Danté in fact was presenting a model of spiritual discovery remarkably in line with the Taoist view of the universe as an interpenetrating field of living energy.

Clinically, the authors have utilized the Dantéan concepts of guiding wisdom and the illumination of energetic reality as ways to help patients along the spiritual journey. The first concept – guiding wisdom – is identical to Assagioli's concept of the Higher Self. Psychosynthetic techniques related to the Higher Self activate the innate centre of guiding wisdom in the patient. Illumination of energetic reality is not within the standard psychosynthetic methods, but Assagioli's model of consciousness is clearly an energy model: in his undated archived notes he has this bold notation: "In India, God was Mind, Consciousness. In Christianity, Love is emphasised. But God is energy, and the religion of the next century will be the study of energy".

To assist patients in exploring the energetic realm of reality, the authors have incorporated Qigong methods in their practice. The methods are applied in the psychosynthetic attitude of an open, scientifically-minded exploration of the spiritual dimension of human nature. Assagioli clearly sets the standard for this attitude: "...we hope to see developed...a science of the Self, of its energies, its manifestations, of how these energies can be released, how they can be contacted, how they can be utilized for...therapeutic work" (1965, p. 194).

The patient's spiritual search may go in many directions over the course of his life. The psychosynthetic therapist can be the one who, as Assagioli put it, "leads the person to the door" (*ibid*).

Summary

The following steps summarize a psychosynthetic approach to the addictive process and the path of recovery:

1 Addiction is an obsessive-compulsive cycle driven by the need to suppress vulnerability.
2 All people are vulnerable, but people who feel a greater degree of vulnerability are drawn to addiction as a remedy.
3 The first step in recovery from addiction is detoxification. Then psychoeducation and psychotherapy are possible.
4 The first task in psychoeducation and psychotherapy is the building of a sober sub-personality.
5 Since the addiction was suppressing vulnerability, the end of addiction will cause vulnerability to be a primary problem again. People in recovery begin to heal by recognizing and respecting their vulnerability.
6 The patient's continued recovery is based on developing new, healthier responses to vulnerability.
7 This vulnerability, however, cannot be effectively responded to on a long-term basis by the ego level of the self, since the ego-level of self is at the very root of vulnerability.
8 Advanced recovery therefore requires the development of an expanded, spiritual sense of identity. Such spiritual development is a normal aspect of adult development.
9 Psychosynthesis offers insights and practices that can introduce the patient to their innate spiritual dimension.

The treatment of addictions is a complex process but well worth the effort. Even in the many frustrations of dealing with people in recovery, the therapist should remember this single point: addiction can be completely cured. People can lead the rest of their lives without addiction. The therapist gets the opportunity to participate with the patient in the transformation of suffering into a purposeful life.

References

Alcoholics Anonymous, *Alcoholics Anonymous: The Big Book*, Alcoholics Anonymous World Services, 1976, 3rd ed

Alcoholics Anonymous, *Twelve Steps and Twelve Traditions*, 1952.

Assagioli R, *Psychosynthesis*, Penguin Books, New York, 1965

Assagioli R, 'The Balance and Synthesis of the Opposites', *Psychosynthesis Research Foundation*, 1975

Danté, *Inferno*, Penguin Books, 1984

Schaub, B and Schaub, R, *Danté's Path*, Penguin Books, 2003

Schaub, B and Schaub, R, *Healing Addictions*, Delmar, 1997

The Silenced Call of Self

Theo Dijkman

Our birth is but a sleep and a forgetting:
The Soul that rises with us, our life's Star,
Hath had elsewhere its setting,
And cometh from afar
(Wordsworth)

Introduction

For over 22 years I have worked with survivors of childhood sexual abuse both in various roles within the third sector and as a psychotherapist. Many excellent books have been written on the impact of childhood abuse and how to work with this within psychotherapy. It is not my intention to focus on how to work with survivors of childhood abuse. Instead I would like to focus on how the relationship between I and Self is silenced through early life trauma and how this has an impact at a psycho-spiritual level.

The Call of Self

Not in entire forgetfulness,
And not in utter nakedness,
But trailing clouds of glory do we come
From God, who is our home:
Heaven lies about us in our infancy!
(Wordsworth)

Eighteen months ago Maisie was born and I became a grandfather. The day after her birth I went to visit my daughter and her newborn and saw a proud mother gaze at this little bundle of life bringing joy. Over the next few days many visitors came and I saw the generosity, love and goodness that Maisie brought into the world. She was given presents knitted by the grandmothers of children my wife taught and who would never see her. The house was filled with the harmony between my daughter and her partner and everyone who visited could feel the warmth and love both from the wood burning stove and the overall atmosphere in the house.

Love created Maisie and Maisie generated love as she came into this world. Love is one of the qualities of Self, one of the many transpersonal qualities that link us both with spirit and others. Tielhard de Chardin suggested that we are not human beings having a spiritual experience, we are spiritual beings having a human experience and birth is the start of our human journey. Assagioli wrote about the 'I', or the self in the world, being a reflection of Self, that unmoving essence of life. Personality is formed around this 'I' obscuring or making us forget our true essence. From the moment of incarnation we start to forget that we are spirit born into matter. Assagioli mentioned that we are as much driven by our search for wholeness, our search for re-connection with Self, as seeking to heal our history. At birth and in our early years of development we do not have the level of consciousness to be aware of this search for Self. Later as we grow up and develop a more refined level of consciousness we may experience this search for wholeness as a vague sense that we are here for a reason.

Assagioli mentioned that "Self is where we come into contact with Mystery, with the supreme Reality, it is outside the confines of science and psychology" (1993, p. 31). We can use words to point at Self, we can give Self many different names, but ultimately Self is beyond description. He also suggested that there are in fact no two selves, no 'I' in the world and Self beyond. Our experience is one of duality, of being split, separate from the other, from Self, yet Self is universal. "The universal Self gives us a sense of permanence and stability and this sense is transmitted from the spiritual Self to its counterpart, the conscious 'I'" (Assagioli, 1993, p. 30). At a personal level the "essential characteristic of self-awareness is continuity and permanence, yet at a personal level that self-awareness of the conscious 'I' is but a poor reflection of the enduring, immortal essence of the Self" (Assagioli, 1993, p. 30).

So while we are spiritual beings on a human journey what many of us can experience is feeling separated, alone and not part of spirit. We can feel separated from the world around us, our loved ones, our relations at work, or from our friendships where we do not truly feel connected and we can feel separated from purpose, meaning and values in our lives. We feel lost as to what we are in the world for, separated in fact from our Self.

Wordsworth wrote about this forgetting of our origin in his Ode of Immortality. As I understand the poem he expressed the idea that as the child grows into adulthood its priority shifts under the influence of its care givers from being connected to the wonder and joy of Self to focussing on worldly matters. In this we fall asleep to our divinity and yet he also expressed that we can re-experience moments of being connected to a deeper meaning in life.

This echoes Assagioli who mentioned that in our day to day life we are limited and restricted and often slaves to our own fantasies and complexes. It can often feel that we are tossed about between conflicting thoughts and emotions and because of this we can feel insecure and not at ease. We experience a split where we feel intuitively that we are one yet we find that we are divided unto ourselves. Yet we can also experience moments where we are lifted out of our ordinary experience and reconnect again with Self.

Joan Evans called this experience of being split a sacred wound. She mentioned that it is the soul which suffers separation and limitation and that this starts from the moment of incarnation.

"The soul is the medium of experience storing memory of the Being's incarnation experiences and is the one which suffers 'divine homesickness' which serves to remind the individual of the Whole. This serves to guide the separated spark towards Life and reminds the individual that in that state of separated wholeness he or she is only a part of the Oneness" (Evans, 2009, p. 93).

She added to this: "In the beginning the 'I' goes unconscious to the Self. The 'I', the spark of the Self, is born into matter, symbolised by the womb of the mother, and this is the first and primary relationship. A more-or-less safe haven is experienced within the embrace of the mother." (Evans, 2009, p. 93).

Maisie's birth was a spark of Self being born into matter and through the embrace, both physical and psychological of her mother, she experiences herself. As the months pass she grows and slowly starts to become more able to move about and away from her mother. As her awareness increases day by day she starts to feel that she is separate, from mother, and ultimately from Self, from which she was born.

Ideally we will develop a secure sense of ourselves through our earliest relationships and through this we can function independently in the world. Maisie's venturing out into the corridor and into another room while looking back to see if we are looking at her is helping her to feel both connected and separate. She will be able to hold onto the memory of mother as a secure base that she can always return to and this again will help her to venture further and further away. I would like to add to this that our ability to venture further and further is ideally not just because we can hold our earliest secure environments in mind but in fact we can hold our connection to Self in mind.

Firman and Gila in the Primal Wound (1997) wrote that our connection to Self provides directionality for individual unfoldment and meaningful engagement with the world, which we receive through our care givers who provide us with a sense of continuity of being. The different relationships we have with empathic care givers, teachers and peers allow us to build a sense of continuity of 'I' over time in the world. These relationships help us to form a relationship with both our internal world, Self and the external world.

We are not just spiritual beings, we are also relational beings. Our very first relationship is between the Self and 'I'. From the moment of conception there is also the physical relationship between mother and growing foetus. There is an intimate and direct experience of ourselves at a physical level in the womb. This physical experience of ourselves continues once we are born. Through touch, mother's skin against ours, and all our other senses we begin to experience ourselves relationally. Taste, sight, sound all help us to build a relationship with the world around us. As we grow up we hopefully will become more confident in our bodies, able to walk, swim and cycle, being encouraged and praised for our competencies. These empathic connections give us the strength of selfhood to engage the widest possible range of human experience. This gives us the strength to experience pain as well as joy, anger as well as love, the complete spectrum that is part of being human. Finally these relationships also help us to create a narrative about who we are; we can tell who we are in terms of our chronological experience through relationships with others. As we grow and develop over time we shape our beliefs, values and worldview.

So through our physicality and different relationships, Self calls us to remember who we truly are; spiritual beings on a human journey. We can also hear the call of Self in the solitude and different sounds in nature, as Wordsworth wrote. We can find it when we are touched by beautiful music, art and in ecstatic religious experiences. We can say that Self continuously tries to draw our attention, flirts with us. Self also calls us at times of crises and change when we consider what direction we want to take in life. One way to consider crises is that they occur when a different level of consciousness is needed, when in fact Self calls to lift our understanding to a different level. Existential questioning, searching for purpose and meaning in life are all part of the call of Self.

How the call of Self is silenced

Whither is fled the visionary gleam?
Where is it now, the glory and the dream?
(Wordsworth)

We have at our disposal many different mechanisms to ignore, or silence the call of Self. The experience of the sacred wound can lead us to splitting off certain aspects of ourselves, our feelings and parts of our awareness. In this we silence or go silent to the call of Self and it is my intention to consider the different strategies or mechanisms that we have at our disposal for this silencing to happen. In what follows I would like to focus on the particular psycho-spiritual wounding caused by childhood abuse, what we can call soul trauma.

In addition to the sacred wound with which we enter the world there is a secondary wounding caused by breaks in the empathic connection with our care givers. Firman and Gila called this secondary wounding the primal wound. They wrote that the break in empathic connection can lead to experiencing non-being energies. They suggested that we are dependent on the other to affirm and experience that we exist. Where there is no empathic connection with these early environments or where this is seriously disrupted we experience a threat to being. They proposed that this threat of non-being is more terrible than death itself. To avoid the extreme feelings associated with this dread, we turn to mechanisms and behaviours that seem to give respite from these feelings. In other words we can dissociate from our experience of ourselves, and in this, break or silence the connection with Self.

Let us consider for a minute how childhood sexual abuse impacts both on everyday living and the connection to Self. The following case study is informed by the experiences of a number of different clients I have worked with.

• • •

The client is a single mother of two children, a young boy and a daughter of 13. She herself is in her thirties and has been in a number of relationships with men, but now lives alone. She was abused in her early teens by two different PE teachers and at the time was not able to tell anyone about it as the men had threatened her that they would also abuse her sister if she did. As time went by and she grew older it became difficult to disclose the abuse to her parents as she didn't want to hurt them, did not want to make them feel that they had not been there for her. On one occasion in her early twenties she had spoken to a friend about what had happened. The friend had looked shocked, was horrified and had insisted that she should go to the police. She couldn't make herself do this, was terrified of what would happen.

She has always hated all physical activities as it made her think about what happened. She has struggled with her weight and does not like the way her body looks. She has periods of binge eating and sticking to strict diets, or making herself sick after she has eaten too much.

Despite having two children she used to find it hard to be physically close to men. In the past she would always have a good drink to help her relax on a night out and family and friend always thought that she was easy going. They don't understand why she does not go out anymore. She blames herself that her children's fathers left because she hated being touched by them or having sex with them and was not surprised that they went looking for someone else.

She has now become more and more isolated, stays in more and hardly dares to go out even to do the shopping. Her family blames her for being difficult and friends have given up on her.

She loves her children dearly but blames herself for letting them down as she is not taking them out much or going on holidays. She is very protective towards them, particularly her daughter who is now getting into her teens and is starting to argue more and more with her. When the girl wants to go out to meet her friends in the evening she has found it impossible to tell her why she can't and she is now worried that her daughter will do things behind her back.

She does not like crowded places or being physically close to people and avoids using public transport during rush hour or going to large supermarkets. She finds being in busy waiting rooms very difficult and on a number of occasions has walked out of doctors' appointments. Her anxiety gets worse when she can't sit somewhere facing a door or with an easy way to get out. She has had periods of self-harming, cutting herself in her genital area and has not been able to get medical treatment for this as she was not sure she would see a female doctor. She hates to open cans of fizzy juice or see tooth paste squeezed out of a tube. All reminders of the abuse she has experienced.

On the few occasions where she has had physical examinations such as during her pregnancy she has been very anxious. She has been very reluctant to change into hospital gowns and even when the changing cubicle can be locked she has been extremely anxious that someone can come in.

• • •

While Self calls us to become most fully ourselves, where our life is an expression of higher qualities and where we are at ease in our inner being, trauma has the opposite effect. It can be said that we all suffer trauma. Birth itself is a traumatic process and we all experience empathic failures as we grow and develop. This, however, is exacerbated for survivors of childhood sexual abuse as there are additional factors that enforce the silencing.

More often than not the abuser is known to the victim, either as a person in a position of trust, the child's care giver, a teacher, or an older peer. These are all early figures who ideally would enable the child to build a good sense of itself over time. Figures who would enable the growing and developing child to connect to self-worth, trust in self and other and an experience of being loved and being able to love. The perpetrator threatens the child that if they were to talk about what had happened, they would not be believed, they would be punished because they had done something bad or wrong. They may even have threatened that it would affect the relationships they have with those they love, that they might be taken into care. Children who have been abused grow up with a conflicting mix of feelings that most find hard to share with those who could have supported them. There is a real sense of isolation, a silencing of their experience. In protecting her younger sister, as well as her parents' feelings my client had internalised her experience. Not being able to make sense of this she became confused in relation to herself psychologically, 'I am to blame and I hate my body', and was unable to stay connected to that enduring essence Assagioli spoke about. For her there was no continuity of being, instead her life was dominated by terror, where there were endless reminders of the abuse and a constant battle with herself as a product of her history rather than all that she could be.

As a society we have found it hard to acknowledge that abuse takes place. Institutions have failed to look into or have actively suppressed the revelation of abuse. At a more basic level many of us wince when we hear what has happened to young children. So even when it is disclosed and spoken about we can shy away from it. My client's friend, although sympathetic and trying to understand, was shocked to hear what had happened. Like many of us she found it hard to imagine that people could do this to vulnerable beings. Letting in the thought of abuse can be extremely unsettling even when we wish to support the individual who has been affected by this. In this the survivor of abuse receives a message that it is better not to talk about the abuse, to remain silent. My client's struggle with not being able to disclose what had happened to her kept her bound to her history and in this her ability to listen to the call of Self was silenced.

Assagioli wrote that (our) "spiritual development is a long and arduous journey …through strange lands full of surprises, difficulties and even dangers. It involves a drastic transmutation of the 'normal' elements of the personality, an awakening of potentialities hitherto dormant, a raising of consciousness to new realms, and a functioning along a new inner dimension" (1993, p. 39).

Childhood sexual abuse freezes the personality into a land filled with danger, where potentialities remain dormant and where consciousness is not raised to new realms or a new inner dimension of functioning is not achieved. This is what makes childhood sexual abuse a psycho-spiritual wounding.

The Silenced Call of Self

We will grieve not, rather find
Strength in what remains behind;
In the primal sympathy
Which having been must ever be
(Wordsworth)

We started by looking at conception and birth as the beginning of Self in the world. Over time as we develop we become aware of a sense of illusory separation of Self. Yet deep within us we can hear Self calling, it draws our attention and listening to this call enables us to be most fully ourselves. Yet, our experience from early in life can be one of being separated, split off and this has been described as a sacred wound. The sacred wound of incarnation.

Over time we can experience a secondary wounding which is the primal wound of the threat of non-being caused either intentionally or unintentionally through the actions of those around us. Childhood sexual abuse carries a threat to the continuity of being and our response to traumatic experiences can be a further splitting off or dissociation from the feelings that arise from the trauma.

This combined sacred and primal wounding can lead to further defence mechanisms and behaviours that have helped us to survive in the world but can in fact reinforce the silencing of the call of Self. We can therefore speak of childhood abuse in terms of a psycho-spiritual wounding or soul trauma. The work with survivors of abuse from a psychosynthesis perspective is not only about healing the trauma of past relationships but the re-establishing of the relationship with Self.

References

Assagioli, R, *Transpersonal Development – The Dimension Beyond Psychosynthesis*, Thorsons, 1993

Assagioli, R, *Psychosynthesis*, Thorsons, 1993

Teilhard de Chardin. Available from www.en.wikiquote.org

Evans, J, *Core Principles of Psychosynthesis Psychology*, Anamcara Press, 2009, Vol 2

Firman, J and Gila, A, *The Primal Wound – A Transpersonal View of Trauma, Addiction, and Growth*, State University of New York Press, 1997

Wordsworth, W, 'Ode' (Intimations of Immortality From Recollections of Early Childhood) – *Poetry of the English-speaking World*, Heinemann, 1950

The Craft of Psychosynthesis

Will Parfitt

If I speak in the tongues of men or even of angels, but have not love, I am only a discordant gong or a noisy cymbal. (Corinthians 1-13)

During life we go through different developmental stages each marked by a specific transition. There are different ways to describe this, but one of the simplest uses common terms thus:

- [Birth]: experience of birth passage
- Baby: transition: turning over and crawling
- Toddler: transition: standing up and walking
- Child: transition: puberty
- Teenager: transition: leaving home
- Young adult: transition: becoming responsible
- Mature adult: transition: integration (and disintegration)
- Elder: letting go
- [Death]

Each healthy transition inevitably involves three steps, helpfully defined by Murray Stein (1983, p. 42) as: separation, liminality, return. Clients often enter psychotherapy when a new transition is immanent and they are resisting the changes, when in transition already and dealing with the lure of the past or fear of the future, or when entering a new stage and needing support in finding their way in their 'new life'.

For instance, consider an individual moving from being a young to mature adult. Let's assume she has relatively successfully passed through the previous transitional phases, has left home and is living the life of a young adult, and is reasonably contented. Then the 'pressures' of the next phases start being felt as she becomes aware there may be more to life than the young adult's carefree life-for-the-moment attitude. As with all of life's transitional phases, this can cause crises of various kinds but all underpinned by a resistance to change and the difficulties this may bring. Our young woman wants things to stay as they are, but as she enters into the transition deeper factors come into play. Unfinished or unresolved matters from previous stages and transitions in her life journey come to the fore once again. A deeply felt desire may emerge not only for life to remain the same but to be able to revert to a previous stage that may now be perceived as simpler and happier. "If only I could still be a child looked after by mum", she might feel, even if not willing to consciously acknowledge such an idea with its attendant feelings of shame and failure. At the same time there is a call from the future, an evolutionary imperative to move on in life and start to take more responsibility. In this example, this imperative may emerge, for instance, as a desire to settle and raise a family, or to more deeply enter into the intricacies of a career. It may simply be to be more deeply engaged with the ups and downs of life.

Assagioli, in drawing the Egg Diagram with dotted lines to stress that the boundaries between different stages and levels of our psyche are not fixed but continuously permeable, shows how our past is not simply personal and individual but also archetypal, ancestral and collective. Dealing with current life transitions can be therefore further complicated by the 'input' into our psyche from all these other influences. Not pushing too soon or trying to create artificial resolution to past or current transitional situations, but watching for opportunities to invoke potential is an important part of the psychosynthesis approach to such situations. This may simply be holding a sense of the importance for a client of uncovering their next step or steps in life.

This is all rather academic, however, for a client who is embroiled in the challenges and difficulties of being in transition, learning to recognize and honour the importance of liminality, the crossroads on the far edge or margin of what had previously seemed an immutable reality. To step into the threshold of the new may involve a kind of initiation, but a typical client is far too engaged with the inherent issues of being at a crossroads to be concerned with niceties of meaning and understanding. They just want to feel better, or at least have a safe place to reflect on both their past and their potential, and most importantly to stay aware of what they are experiencing in the present situation. This is often frightening – there are no structures to help stabilize them as energies from the depths of the psyche are emerging, often chaotically. As Murray Stein (1983, p. 41) commented when defining liminality, they have entered "the condition in which ego becomes unmoored from its former fixities of identification and identity and 'floats'..."

With the therapist's help the client has to 'get real' and overcome the pretence that life is controllable and manageable. The 'old' has to die to make space for the 'new' and a psychosynthesis therapist will help clients find inner resources to go through this death and re-birth experience without in any way avoiding or denying the dangers involved. Crossings are dangerous, there's no doubt about that, but they also offer opportunities.

To be able to work at this effectively, the therapist must also deeply reflect on both what is and what is not comfortable in their own life: what are they identified with, attached to in their life; what makes them comfortable and secure and what they are bonded or attached to in order to get that security, and whether this is enough. Such deep reflection inevitably includes what frustrates, constricts, holds them in bondage – to put it bluntly, what is missing when they are 'safe at home' at whatever stage of development they are at in their life journey. A therapist can be most effective in their work if they ask such questions of themselves and are willing to be face to face with the perennial dilemma of the old being outworn whilst the new is uncertain. He or she can then hold a client in the uncertainty, not rushing to force entry through the door of the new but staying with awareness in the liminal.

If as therapists we are being asked to work in liminality, then a question we have to ask is what kind of people hang out at crossroads, on borders, and in other such liminal spaces? On the negative side, we mostly think of highwaymen, robbers, and other questionable and dangerous entities that feed on peoples' difficulties, even vampires of the psychic if not literal type. There are also often guards who won't (or can't) just let you go through unless you have the right credentials. On the more positive side, we find explorers, guides, and individuals who have chosen to serve those in such dangerous crossing places. As well as psychotherapists we often find witches and magicians, people who identify themselves as occultists and often describe their path as 'the craft', the underlying intention of which is to know oneself. Psychosynthesis psychotherapists have the same intention: using the 'craft' of uncovering what has been previously covered or hidden to aid clients come to know themselves.

The techniques used by psychotherapists and occultists in their respective crafts initially appear different, but delving below the surface we find this may not be so obviously the case. Craft is not about techniques, it is not the content of a training, it is not the obvious. It is not being a Gardnerian Witch, an adept of the Golden Dawn, or a graduate of a specific psychosynthesis course. To engage the craft means to be 'crafty', to see the 'something else' that is inherent in everything, the deeper 'soul' or 'meaning' which brings insight and understanding.

A magician's craft is based on a grimoire (a book of magic spells) which is the grammar of this language, and the words used are those of 'spell'-ing. A therapist's craft is what is learned in a training that does *not* fit into the prospectus: it is the stuff of dreams and myths, of relationship and presence.

A magician works in a temple, the external universe as it is found. This corresponds to the therapy room and the previously unexplored territory of the new client's psyche. In this temple a circle is drawn upon the floor to define the limitations of the work, to create a container and to announce the nature of the Great Work (of 'knowing oneself'.) The circle is the appropriate boundaries the therapist keeps, and the vessel (or 'field') in which the work of relationship unfolds. The circle is protected by divine names (the therapist's ethics and own oath to Self).

All craft has tools to make it visible and effective. Within a magical circle stands an altar, which is described as the solid base or foundation of the work. It is the past experience of the client (and the therapist), upon which all the work is inevitably based, and which offers a ground or base for understanding. Upon the altar are a wand for will, a cup for love, a sword for reason and a pentacle which represents the body.

A magician uses oil which consecrates everything it touches and represents aspiration. In the therapeutic container it is the joint aspiration of the therapist and client, working together to create a new future (which allows for the presence of soul). A magician also uses a scourge to excite sluggish nature (challenge), a dagger which calms too great a heat (support), and a chain to bind the wandering thoughts (focused attention). These keep the aspirations pure.

Above the altar hangs a light, representing the light of pure soul. It is a reminder not to be too confident or clever, that something in the craft is always unknown and beyond ('...and I am more than this'.) For the therapist it is a reminder to honour the divinity of the client. A magician also wears a crown (to affirm his or her divinity), a single robe (to symbolize silence and protection) and over the heart a special seal (to remind the practitioner that the secret keys of power and love are found in the heart.) A magician carries a magical record or journal (both the personal journal of the therapist and the client notes), and a bell (which summons and alarms). For the therapist the clock is the reminder of the passage of time – it summons the hour's end and can be a timely reminder of the impermanence of all things.

Jack Parsons (1980, p. 33), a magician and founder of the Jet Propulsion Laboratory, wrote: "The way we show is not easy; it is hard because to know one's self is always hard. To break through the shell of the little world and undo the hypnotization of generations is difficult. We have no soothing syrup..." (1980) and, later; "in fairy tales and playing cards, in myths and legends, in strange poems and old songs, we hid the secret knowledge. Now and then an adventurer into dark ways and lonely lands of the soul has come amazed upon the 'pearl of great price'" (*ibid*). That pearl is the craft embodied; it is the Great Work, the work of the heart.

Inevitably such work requires the invention of a new therapy for each client, remembering all the while that difficulty equals opportunity. All individuals experiencing separation, liminality or re-integration require careful handing and individual attention. For instance, a psychosynthesis therapist might be concurrently exploring with a client issues from their past, for example mystic, victim and rebel subpersonalities, disconnections in the client's present experience, and his or her fears for their future.

One metaphor used to understand the intention of the more negative people that hang out at crossroads is that they want to interfere with or even capture the soul of those who find themselves there in transitional crisis. To some psychotherapists this might sound a rather fanciful description but it does have a traditional connection in shamanic soul retrieval work. Of course, once we start using the word 'soul' we enter into the area of opinion and debate. What is soul and can we even be sure we have one? Indeed, even in religious traditions that apparently assert the inevitable presence of soul this is not necessarily the truth. Jacob Needleman (1990, p. 176) describes a search for the meaning of soul that leads him to discover a hidden and original idea in early (and current Greek Orthodox) Christianity that we are not born with soul but have to grow it. "It was a disaster for Christianity when it adopted the notion that the soul of man already exists in finished form within human nature. This assumption about the given existence of soul led to our identification of ordinary kinds of thoughts, emotions and sensations with the soul...and hence to futile and mistaken efforts to perfect our being by perfecting our thoughts, emotions or sensations."

So whether we are talking literally or metaphorically, we can understand the work of a therapist to be to help clients find their 'soul presence' (that they have or can 'grow a soul'). In psychosynthesis training, students are usually introduced to the notion of bifocal vision, that whilst paying attention to a client's perceptions, sensations and emotions that constitute their ordinary, everyday experience, the therapist also 'keeps an eye on' the higher, freer presence within and behind all, a presence found not only in the client's heights of experience but also in their depths and despair, not only in the light but also in the dark.

To this aim, the therapist becomes an external unifying centre for the client, temporarily taking the role of the client's own centered self and holding this strongly enough to allow the client not only to go into their depth but also to face their heights or potential. The underlying intent is always to give back this centre to the client, to help re-introduce this centered presence within them. As Firman and Gila express it: "Furthermore, as each stage of life is supported and held by the appropriate, empathic, external unifying centre, the active interaction with that external unifying center conditions the formation of an inner representation or inner model of that center – an internal unifying center" (2002, p 119).

The idea is to encourage the inner unifying centre in the client by temporarily embodying his or her external centre. The main focus is to stay with what is in the present encounter, invite the presence of the Self, and trust that what needs to will emerge. A useful perspective is to focus on changing motivation to intention in a soft, 'crafty' way so the motivating energy that brought the client to therapy (the painful and unpleasant experience) is transformed into a self-responsible intent. This is sometimes rather simplistically expressed as changing the 'I won't' to an 'I will'. Then 'when the heart weeps for what it has lost, the spirit laughs for what is has found' in the old Sufi saying.

Psychosynthesis psychotherapists can be seen as alchemists, working to discover the universal solvent that will 'turn lead to gold' or transform the mundane into the 'elixir of life'. In therapeutic terms this can be understood as a great shift (or 'alchemy') from being centered on the belly, a victim to tides of emotions, uncontrollable thoughts, fears, fantasies, unfulfillable wishes, and so on, to being centered on the heart. In the psychosynthesis Egg Diagram, the individual self is placed at the centre just as, energetically, the heart is the natural centre of the human system. The therapist holding an external unifying centre for a client intends returning heart to the client or in other words, retrieving their soul. This is underpinned by the belief that psyche has its own inherent healing energy and wants to centre on heart. Assagioli, in defining psychosynthesis, asserted that it is: "A method that… helps (the individual) to discover and realize his true spiritual nature, and to build under its guidance a harmonious, radiant and efficient personality" (1975, p. 30).

The therapist helps the client identify and deal with obstacles in the way of this path, following the basic Rogerian principles of congruence, empathy and, most importantly, unconditional positive regard. By remaining heart centered in this way, the therapist learns he or she is not there to do anything else and, in fact, doing anything else may well be counter-productive (even in short term counselling.) This approach does not de-skill the therapist, but rather it aims to empower the client in a relationship that is inevitably intersubjective. The elixir of life (the production of which is the aim of the therapeutic alchemy) is then simply and clearly the effect of unconditional love in a relationship.

A therapeutic encounter consists of two distinct subjective realities and the space or field between them. Jung expressed it as "a state of mystical participation full of uncertainty and creative chaos" (quoted in Whitmore, 1991, p. 121). Psychosynthesis therapists are therefore exhorted to not give up their techniques and understanding but to free up space for these to function craftily without the obstacles they themselves may bring to the meeting, mainly egoism and preconceptions. This then engenders a transformative environment. After all, the non-participating objective therapist is a myth: we can't hide our unconscious messages, they are revealed through body and speech, so to carefully explore the present, 'here and now' relationship is always the essence of the work. Just as those who identified themselves with the Craft in days gone by were part of an ongoing tradition, psychosynthesis therapists can position themselves similarly, aware that their work is in line with the perennial wisdom and central to the Great Work of alchemy, to know oneself individually, intersubjectively and collectively.

References

Assagioli, R, *Psychosynthesis*, Turnstone Books, 1975

Firman, J and Gila, A, *Psychosynthesis: A Psychology of the Spirit*, SUNY Press, 2002

Jung, CJ, *Development of the Personality*, Princetown University Press, 1954

Needleman, J, *Lost Christianity*, Elements Books Ltd, 1990

Parsons, J, *The Witchcraft*, 93 Publishing, 1980

Stein, M, *In Midlife*, Spring Publications Inc., 1983

Soulmaking at Work

I am Self

Harry Jenkins

About five years ago my spiritual path turned to non-duality. The non-duality teaching centres on an exploration of consciousness and asks who we are most essentially. It looks outwards at our consciousness of the world and inwards at our interior experiences such as thinking and feeling. Retreats and meetings have a similar atmosphere to training weekends in psychosynthesis and the teaching is very compatible. Non-duality has allowed me to deepen my understanding of the Self.

In this paper I wish to share that deeper understanding by discussing the Self and to a lesser extent, the 'I'. (I shall use 'I' with quotation marks to mean the psychosynthesis 'I' and I without quotation marks to mean the common usage of the word I in day to day conversation.) I start by setting the scene with a very brief discussion of the 'I' and the Self. Afterwards, I take us through a thought experiment intended to bring a direct experiential experience of the Self. I do this by introducing what I am going to call awareness and then show that this awareness is another name for the Self. I finish with some thoughts on how this affects therapy.

What are the Self and the 'I' in psychosynthesis? "The Transpersonal Self is an *ontological reality*, a *being* and is on its own level a stable Centre of Life, from which it radiates energies. The *personal* self, the self-conscious 'I', is a projection or reflection of the Self into the normal human level" (Evans, 2003, p. 166). "The Self has a sense of identity based on the pure awareness of being and unity with the All. Its very essence is consciousness free of all contents, beyond time and cultural conditioning…It has a serene, broad perspective, originating in a cosmic viewpoint… possibly the deathless nucleus of each human being" (Ferrucci, 1990, p. 342).

Assagioli, speaking of the Self and 'I' in the context of the Egg Diagram, states it like this: "There are not really two selves, two independent and separate entities.

The Self is one; it manifests in different degrees of awareness and self-realisation. The reflection appears to be self-existent but has, in reality, no autonomous substantiality. It is, in other words, not a new and different light but a projection of its luminous source" (1990 p. 20).

The Self infuses the Egg, but also the world outside of the Egg. Everything within the Egg or outside the Egg is made of the Self. The Self is pure consciousness. It is the only ontological reality. The 'I' is a case of the Self misidentifying itself with limitation and encasement in a body, of apparently being less than it truly is.

At this point I need to define two words which I want to use: consciousness and awareness. Both these words have a specific meaning in psychosynthesis which I would like you to put to one side for the time being. Instead, I invite you to temporarily think of awareness as it is often used colloquially in conversations. The Oxford Dictionary of English (2005) defines aware as: having knowledge or perception of a situation or fact; and awareness as the associated noun, the state of being aware. Furthermore, I am not using awareness to mean *having* thoughts, but the state of being aware of thoughts. Awareness is contentless. I will use consciousness as a synonym *of* awareness. In addition, I will also use 'know' as a synonym for 'aware'. For instance, I do not use 'know' in the sense of: I know my two times table, meaning I have internalised knowledge of the table. Rather I mean that I know or observe a series of thoughts occurring: one two is two, two twos are four, etc.

'I' is aware, or as we might say, conscious. It "is the inner experience of pure self-awareness, independent of any content or function of the ego in the sense of personality" (Assagioli 1990, p. 112). It is the awareness defined above, but overlaid with an identification as a separate self. 'I' is the Self dressed in the clothes of separation, taking itself to be an individual consciousness, contained in a body, moving around in a material world. It is apparently limited by believing itself to be within a body and a mind. It believes that there are around 7 billion separate consciousnesses on this planet, ignoring animals, and that it is one of these. It experiences more peace than a subpersonality, but it is not a peaceful experience to live like this as 'I' experiences inevitable conflicts with other 'I's and fears death.

I turn now to a train of thought, which if you take the time to check out in your own experience could lead to a direct experience of Self. Let us start with how the word I is used in normal conversation when someone says for instance, "I work as a psychotherapist". People tend to mean the corporeal body, their thoughts or feelings when they say I. As psychosynthesis practitioners we are clear that we are not only our body, mind or feelings. So, what or who are we?

We can note from experience that we are aware of the body, thoughts and feelings. In fact, if we close our eyes, our only experience of a body is sensation, such as the tingling in our legs. Without turning to memories of our body image there is nothing else that we know in that moment. Experientially, this seemingly solid body is only ever known directly as sensations. Even if we open our eyes, we will see a small part of what we take to be our body, but even this is only known as perception or seeing. We never actually know an independent solid body.

Similarly, if we pay attention to thoughts we can notice that their only existence is in the awareness of them. Try as we might, we can never find a thought with a separate existence to the awareness of it. Turning our attention to feelings, we discover the same thing. We can never find a feeling with a separate existence to the knowing of it. Knowing seems to be an inextricable part of all experiences.

We could use other words for knowing. One would be experiencing and another, as I previously said, awareness. Sensations (the body), thoughts and feelings are only ever known through or as awareness.

When we disidentify from thoughts, feelings and sensations we identify with what knows them, namely with awareness. This awareness is a deeper and truer statement of who we are. We are awareness. We can never be objects that come and go. We know deep down that we are always present, not coming and going as thoughts or sensations come and go.

As we look closer, we realise that awareness is at the heart of all perceptions too. By perceptions I mean seeing, hearing, tasting, touching and smelling. It is by perceptions that we know the world outside of us. In fact, without perceptions we would know nothing of a world. If you look now to find something that you are not aware of, you cannot do it. At best, you can think of or imagine that thing, but can never find it directly without the tools of perception.

We have learned since first childhood that we are separate from the world we perceive, and many of us believe ourselves to be our thoughts, our feelings, our body or all three. However, as we disidentify from these interior experiences to being awareness only, we notice that our internal world and the exterior world are both equally known by this awareness. From awareness's viewpoint, there is no meaningful difference. Everything is known or experienced.

Take a moment to ask yourself, 'Am I aware?' We all know without doubt that we are aware. It is not something that we need to work out intellectually, but a deep knowing. In fact, it is the only certainty. Everything that we experience could be false, perhaps a hallucination, but the one certainty in all cases is that we are aware. Even when we dream, awareness is at the heart of the dream for without it the dream would never be known.

I am aware. I am awareness. We now have another name for awareness as well as knowing or experiencing, and that name is I. I am not my body, my thoughts or my feelings. Rather, I am awareness.

When we explore awareness, or in other words ourself, we discover that we can make some definite statements about ourself. Firstly, we can find no limits to awareness/ourself. Secondly, we notice that we are present. We are not elsewhere or in some way not present. Thirdly, nothing is ever known, or could ever be known, that does not appear in or to awareness.

Ideally, we would disidentify to awareness by transcending and including thoughts, feelings, sensations (the body) and perceptions of the world. Unfortunately, and almost inevitably, the first step to standing as awareness is one of discarding everything known by claiming that these things (objects) are not me. At this point, we would stand as awareness, aware of a myriad of internal and external objects. We would feel apart from the maelstrom, in a place of pure peace. In spiritual circles this is sometimes known as the Witness position. Note that this is not a subpersonality, just as the psychosynthesis 'I' and Self are not.

The typical next step on this spiritual journey is to realise that I am not contained in a body or mind, but rather that the body and mind appear in me. In other words, all experiences of anything whatsoever appear in or to awareness. This step to stand as the Witness imagines awareness as pure subjectivity aware of all thinking, feeling, sensing and perceiving. The Witness takes itself to be apart from experience, a witness of it. This is a step of dissociation. The body/mind/world are all dissociated leaving only awareness or consciousness. It is a place of peace, but is also sterile. The Witness is above the fray and unaffected by it.

What happens next on the spiritual path is extraordinary. Gradually, or sometimes suddenly, we begin to notice that the body/mind/world are not separate from awareness. They are not apart, witnessed from afar, but are made of awareness itself. We have already noticed that no object can be known without awareness of it being involved. What we now come to see is that there are no independent objects. There are no thoughts, feelings, sensations or perceptions. Likewise, there is no thinker, feeler, sensor or perceiver. There is only thinking, feeling, sensing and perceiving. The world and the perceiver collapse into perceiving. Similarly the thought and the thinker collapse into thinking. Moreover, we realise that thinking, feeling, sensing and perceiving are all just different aspects of being aware. There is nothing but awareness. Nothing but consciousness. Nothing but what we mean when we say I.

We realise that we are not a witness of events, we are the very stuff of all life, of all that appears to happen. We are pure being, presence, awareness, unlimited, not many. There is nothing that is not me. We have transcended separation and alienation, yet at the same time include all apparent difference and separation. We no longer have dissociation, but disidentification that transcends and includes. At this point we no longer identify with a separate self meeting other separate selves. There is only awareness, whole and unbroken. The collapse of separation reveals love, happiness and peace in this total intimacy where everything is me. Separation into separate 'I's is revealed to be illusory. There was never anything but awareness, taking the form of separation.

The Self is nothing other than the awareness we have been speaking of, also called consciousness, and named too as the I of conversation once this I is stripped of separation and misidentifications. The Self/awareness is perfect acceptance of all that arises. Awareness, by its very nature can resist nothing. The psychotherapist who takes her or his stand as Self/awareness is open to all that arises in the therapy room. All egoic resistance has dropped away because there is no longer a separate ego with egoic defences present. Moreover, this Self is all that arises, without exception.

Taking your stand as Self requires seeing all that arises as unseparated, an unbroken continuity. Concepts such as I-Thou are transcended by the realisation that in reality there is no I and no Thou, only Self. There are not two Selves, only One. It means letting go of the idea of being a person in here looking at a world out there of separate individuals and objects. There are no separate people or objects, neither you nor others. There is only awareness/consciousness/Self dancing as all that arises with neither an observer nor any thing observed.

Turning to therapy, taking your stand as Self is to see no separation between the apparent therapist and apparent client. Thoughts and feelings arise, but belong to no one. They just are. The tears of the 'client' are your tears. The fear of the 'client' is your fear. The words of the 'client' are your words and the words of the 'therapist' are their words. There is no client and no therapist, just words, thoughts, feelings, sensations and perceptions all arising in perfect harmony. There is nothing to be done and no one to do it. Instead there is total intimacy, without separation, which is love.

Carl Rogers' concept of unconditional positive regard speaks to a similar idea. In other words, he may have intuited, as perhaps did Buber with his concept of I-Thou, that you and I are most essentially one. We can put bi-focal vision in the same category, where what is obvious from the viewpoint of Self is represented in the dual world of separate me speaking to separate you. In practice, treating our client as most essentially ourself is a good way of applying the viewpoint of the Self without letting go of the idea of separate individuals.

Taking the viewpoint of Self, the concept of counter transference can be re-worked. No longer is there a separate client inducing thoughts and feelings in a separate therapist. All thoughts and feelings belong to Self. There is only one consciousness, not two, and it no longer makes sense to talk as though there are separate consciousnesses where one consciousness affects the other. As there is only one Self, the fact of the therapist speaking of a feeling being present and the client acknowledging it makes total sense. It is only the Self expressing itSelf in two different voices.

Working in this way does not take away any of the skills of a psychosynthesis therapist. The wonderings about transference and counter transference still arise and models still remain relevant and potentially illuminating. But instead of an apparently separate therapist taking responsibility for her or his interventions, there is letting go into trust of Self as the source of each intervention. It is the Self that is unfolding during the therapy and whatever appears to happen, the Self remains itSelf, both appearing to take different shapes and forms, yet remaining always and forever itSelf.

Trusting in Self allows the therapist to let go of any possible attachment to outcomes and provides total acceptance of the client just as they are. This total acceptance is in itself healing. It also allows the therapist to accept, think about and make use of all manner of counter transferential thoughts, feelings or bodily sensations without needing to reject any of them as unacceptable to the therapist. Seeing the therapist, client and their interactions as one unbroken expression of

Self allows another possibility. The therapist can usefully think of the unfolding of the therapeutic encounter as one thing, not belonging to anyone. Thinking like this can bring new insights that would be obscured by dividing the encounter into parts owned by the client and therapist separately.

A practical illustration may help make this way of working clearer. The therapist is late and the client is angry as a result. From the viewpoint of the Self there is lateness and anger, but no separate people. Even if defensiveness or feelings of guilt or reciprocal anger arise in the therapist, he/she can look at these as part of the unfolding event, not as something owned by him/her. This place of disidentification can then allow compassion and empathy to arise as well as the possibility to perhaps see a pattern repeated from the client's childhood of a parent being late and the feelings present in both child and parent.

In conclusion, I have attempted to give a taste of the Self by exploring awareness and seeing that it is the same as the Self. The Self is who you are. The Self is not many, but one, without limit. It is not only who we are most essentially as human beings, but there is nothing but Self, nothing but consciousness. Standing as Self is the ultimate disidentification and allows enormous freedom as a therapist, where the work can be held without attachment, but with love.

References

Assagioli, R, *Psychosynthesis – A Manual of Principles and Techniques*, Mandala, 1990

Oxford Dictionary of English, Oxford University Press, 2005

Evans, J, *Fundamentals of Psychosynthesis*, Anamcara Press, 2003

Ferrucci, P, *Inevitable Grace – Breakthroughs in Self-Realisation*, Crucible, 1990

Contemplative Psychosynthesis: a Personal Exploration

Dorothy Firman

Preamble

As I planned this article, I gathered all the books and resources that would help me build this emerging theory of contemplative psychosynthesis. I had stacks of books from the great masters of Eastern and Western traditions. I planned to track psychosynthesis as it has shown up in the field of psychology, proving, yet again, its enormous value. I had a surprise I intended to add, noting where contemplative psychology has made it into a text book that I use to teach graduate students in the field of psychology. Then, I knew, I would tie it all together. It would be grand. It would be thorough. It would be inviting… and maybe even moving.

I played, "And this bit of psychosynthesis theory is contemplative because…" Every piece of theory does, in fact, lend itself to contemplative practice, so no proof needed. I pondered and solved the riddle of what to do with Assagioli's line about psychosynthesis taking us to the doors of the great mystery but not taking us through. (Assagioli, 2000)

I know how to write. I can do this. It is important to the field. I write academic articles frequently. Citation, citation, citation. Grab a quote to validate a point. Reference list as long as the article.

I called on my favorite Contemplative (noun, not adjective) for his resources and he gladly complied.

I watched the snow fall and stared at the books. I didn't go for a walk.

I forced myself to make an outline.

I doubted my capacity to write this article.

I began the internal story of why it didn't make sense to do this article.

I jumped on the ever-present subtext of my need to learn to say no.

I opened up the arena and watched the subpersonalities do battle, some in outright combat, others in serious debate, the weak ones on the side hoping for their voices to be heard.

I felt awful.

Late last night I wrote a note to Steve Simpson (editor of this book) saying sorry, can't do it. Good luck, blah, blah, blah.

In the quiet of the morning, snow falling again, I breathed a little more deeply. I knew there was no right or wrong about this. I took a walk.

Home again, I sat quietly, settled down and in.

My 40 year practice of watching, sitting still or walking, quieting, stepping back and going empty, kicked in. It is, I admit, a raggedy, unconstructed, practice, informed by many traditions: years of Zen; many more years of martial arts practice; mindfulness (Vipassana) training; a much earlier lifetime of Christianity, exoteric and esoteric; a brief foray in my twenties into gurus; and reading, of course, most everything. What I do practice, now, regularly, formally and informally is almost solely informed by psychosynthesis: psychosynthesis contemplative practice.

I have just come to my computer, more peaceful than I have been in some days. I came to check my email. I began to write instead. If you are reading this, I must imagine that over the next days and weeks I will continue to write.

If you are not reading this, it doesn't matter. I found my resting place, in this moment, on this issue. "The great way is easy for those not attached to preferences" (Seng-Ts'an, 2001).

I have a 'psychosynthesis evangelist' subpersonality. She wants to save the world through psychosynthesis. She wants to save psychosynthesis from the tight jaws of psychology. She wants psychosynthesis to be a household word. Her whole professional life has been psychosynthesis. *I have this part of me and I am not this part.* I have an 'academic' subpersonality, building her resume, playing her Professor role, making offering after offering to the gods of higher education, slipping psychosynthesis into their midst all the while. *I am not the academic.* I have a pleaser sub. *I am not that pleaser.*

The resting place I am in (however briefly it may stay) comes from dis-identifying from my subpersonalities and their particular agendas. My 'academic' usually owns the keyboard. My 'psychosynthesis evangelist' finds her place in teaching. My 'pleaser' slips in so often 'I' may not notice her presence, until she says "yes" when the truth is "no".

But right now, they are quiet. I am in my hara, (my belly). My eyes close between thoughts. Awareness and will move with my breath. Purpose guides me. I am imminent in this world, at my computer, aware of the coldness in the room. I am transcendent, more than that, content-less. *I am a center of pure consciousness and will.*

Contemplative Psychosynthesis

The act of contemplation is as old as human history. We exist in a reality, and by nature, we are inclined, when we can, to understand that reality. We are called, as philosophers, theologians, poets, artists, explorers, scientists and every other man, woman and child, to explore and come to terms with both our outer and inner reality. Assagioli reminds us that the "action of one who is endeavouring to perceive inner reality is called 'contemplation' or the 'contemplative state' " (2010, p. 166). We are perhaps all called, in one way or another, to contemplation.

Psychosynthesis contemplative practice comes from within the very theory and practices of psychosynthesis. Whether we follow Assagioli's quiet wisdom and work with exercises he designed, like the Blossoming of the Rose or Evoking Desired Qualities, the daily practice is even more basic. Everything in psychosynthesis points to accessing Self and to the process of Self-realization. Everything.

Psychosynthesis gives us the guiding truth about Self: that it is a center of content-less awareness and will. There you have it. The technology of contemplative practice is designed to take us right there. *Self-identification* "is the inner experience of pure self-awareness, independent of any content or function of the ego..." (Assagioli, 2000, p. 99). This is the invitation to contemplative practice. It is to be the Self that we are that is not ego, not story, not subpersonality, not psychological functions, not the outcome of our past, not the fantasies of our future, not a product of our culture, not a this or a that. And it is a practice. It is a life's practice. It is based, on what I consider to be the defining practice in psychosynthesis: Identification, Disidentification and Self-identification. This is mindfulness. It is meditation. It is practice, seated in full lotus and practice in the heat of an argument. It is the experience of Self, knowing, honouring and accepting all aspects of our own personalities and our world at large and returning to content-less awareness and will. This is the ground.

Psychosynthesis, freed of its relationship to any religion, and equally freed from its primary current modalities in psychotherapy, coaching and education, becomes unto itself a contemplative practice. This practice could be manifest in many ways.

Imagine that you don't know psychosynthesis, in whatever way you know and use it now. You have entered a retreat setting where you are invited to sit comfortably, time taken to share, context set, leader introduced. The next hours are contemplation.

Sit up straight, alert and relaxed, feet on the floor. Breathe into your belly. Notice your thoughts as you settle in. 'I have these thoughts and I am not these thoughts…'

Continually return to 'I am a centre' and allow all content that wants to define that centre to slip easily away. Move to simply 'I am'.

Stay with your breath and the mantra, if you will, of 'I am'.

As our psychosynthesis contemplative retreat moves on, that exercise gets deepened, and personalised as each participant notes their deepest ego based attachments: to roles, to people, to ideas or beliefs, to survival subpersonalities, to preferences. The dis-identification continues, each attending to and dis-identifying from their unique attachments. This clinging is the stuff of ego, protecting itself from all threat.

Become defenceless is the invitation. An old story, with Zen Buddhist roots, tells of the ronin (renegade samurai) running through the village threatening people with his sword. As people flee up the mountain, they warn the old priest to run. The priest continues to sit. The ronin approaches, rage and power in his hands. Sword at the throat of the quiet priest he yells, "Don't you know I have the power to run you through with my sword?" A breath. A moment. A quiet response, "Don't you know I have the power to be run through by your sword?" Lost, then found, the ronin becomes enlightened. All stories, all identifications, all the props of the ego, dropped away.

Who are you, if you are not all of these passing contents of consciousness? All of these semi-autonomous subpersonalities, holding for dear life to their stories? Who are you if you are no one?

We have our stories, our subpersonalities, our thinking, feeling, impulse, imagination. We have our bodies. We have our plans and expectations. We have our attractions and aversions. We have our names and our sex and our religion. They are all the swords we hold so tightly.

'He not busy being born is busy dying' reminds us of the bookends of a life, but also, what we attach to, between those ends: busy-ness. Bob Dylan, sometimes the modern sage, calls it like it is. If we can imagine *defenceless*, can we imagine *quiet? Empty? Slow? Unattached to outcome? Without preference?* Can you feel who you are beyond your story?

But our retreat continues.

Imagine now the blossoming of the rose, from bud to full blossom.

And from this space of just growing like a rose, just evolving in ways known and unknown, unmoored from old themes, sit in the now, as if it were the only now, no past, no future. What qualities of being do you carry that are simply the colour of your rose?

This retreat could go on and on, based solely on the principles, themes and exercises of psychosynthesis. Assagioli's own writing on meditation could guide us: receptive, reflective, creative (2010). His work with images, colours, shapes, visualization could guide us (2000). His work on the will, so very practical, is also an introduction to a spiritual life, a training in contemplation. Never confuse meditation with awareness, only. It is always awareness and will: the functions of Self. The direction to train the will, one of Assagioli's great gifts to us, might be the very next piece of this imagined retreat.

Please now, in the quiet of your presence, take the box of matches in front of you, and with all consciousness and no attachment to outcome, without counting or making designs, simply take each match out of the box. Breathe. Stop now. What pulled at you as you took each match out? What subpersonalities got activated? What psychological functions, pulled towards dominance? What did the monkey mind do with this 'useless' exercise? Take a moment. "I have all of this and I am not this." Notice what it is in you that attempts to take ownership of your consciousness. Then step back. Breathe. Adjust your posture. Let your body's alignment be the container for your emptiness.

Put each match back in the box, without thought or impulse or assessment or trying. Without conversation, without being in the future or the past. Breathe. Just putting matches in a box.

Such a simple act, as Assagioli's 'useless' will exercise (2010), trains us in contemplation. As traditions from time immemorial have done, psychosynthesis offers us help along the way of contemplation. Mantras, koans, symbols, movement, mudras, body alignment, breath, inspiration, direction. Roberto, like any good Teacher, shows us the many paths (and many pitfalls) in developing our contemplative practice.

As our imaginary retreat ends, we are reminded of our practice. Disidentification, Assagioli tells us, "serves also as a technique for acquiring pure self-awareness, the pure sense of self-identity" (2000, p. 62). He invites us over and over to move towards the 'direct experience' of Self, the end point of all contemplative practice. Self: content-less awareness and will. "The mystics of all times and places have realized and expressed the joy and bliss which are inherent in the union of the individual will with the universal will" (Assagioli, 2010, p. 144). And there we glimpse the transpersonal, transcendent nature of contemplative practice. And as we practice day to day, we equally find our contemplative practice anchoring us into the here and now, worldly, imminent, experience of Self. (See Firman and Gila, 2002, for an elaboration of the idea of "transcendence-immanence.")

Inventing one step further in the blossoming of the rose, we might end our retreat.

And watch the rose as its beautiful blossom fades, petals curl up and drop off. Leaves become brown. The barren bush remains, thorns revealed. Has anything changed? With blossoms or without, in summer or winter, roots or branches or flowers? All are the rose. The earth in which it is firmly seated, the sun which nourishes. Is there a rose that is not inevitably part of this larger whole? Even unto its death?

A Little Theory

Though it is tempting to dip into other contemplative practices, from both the East and West, it is enough, for now, to briefly propose a theory of contemplative practice based solely on psychosynthesis. Very briefly.

The 'I', as a reflection of Self, is a center of consciousness and will. It exists in the midst of levels of unconsciousness that span from the lower to the higher. It exists as an internal unifying center (Assagioli, 2000) waiting to be freed from conditioning that overshadows it and ensnares the human being in the power of the personality. The Self exists at all times and each human being directly experiences that Self at some times. Mostly we experience our subpersonalities, the really difficult ones and the really cool, ego supporting, highly functional ones.

Self is available at the kitchen sink, in the middle of the personality's daily life. It exists on the mountaintop, or on the cushion, or in love or peak experience, at the moment of transcendence, when there is no personality left at all. It exists in the dark night of the soul, when the personality has been shattered, when darkness surrounds.

The Call of Self is the reality of Self's eternal presence. And whether we hear it or not in any given moment, Self always calls. Sometimes it is clear. Sometimes it is hard to decipher. Sometimes we hear and ignore. Nonetheless, Self stays. In tracking a life, mine or yours, at whatever age we are now, we can look back through the lens of the many wounds and losses or we can look back through the lens of this very call. Was it ever not there?

Do you remember your favourite childhood game or activity? Hero? Your particular friends? What spaces, in nature or your home you most preferred to inhabit? Can you remember where you found solace? Joy? Inspiration? Your biography, written through the lens of your Unfolding Self (tip of that hat to Molly Brown's *Unfolding Self*, 2004) is a very different story than the one we take to our therapist's office!

The theory, then, is that Self has one purpose and that is to manifest itself as You. And, if my years of studying psychosynthesis are more or less on track, every piece of theory in psychosynthesis points to Self. There is no other work in psychosynthesis, though the winding road towards Self is complex and difficult. Psychosynthesis provides a masterful guidebook.

A Practice

Assagioli's psychological functions map is the ground for this one, hopefully useful, contemplative practice.

Sitting straight, breathing into the hara (belly/dantien), imagine that the center of the star diagram is your belly. Always return to it.

Breathe into your thinking and welcome whatever thoughts appear. Let the thoughts go.

Breathe into your sensations and experience your body fully in this moment. Leave these sensations and return to your breath.

Smile and know your emotional world, as it is. Whatever feelings present, accept them. Return to your smile. Return to your breath.

Notice your desires, in the moment. Let the 'wanting' of impulse and desire be full. And know there is no need to act on the wanting.

Return to the image of the star diagram, centered in your hara. Enrich it with color and depth. And let it go.

Stay with your breath, emptying the space and invite intuition to enter. However it presents, if it presents, hold it, for just a breath, and let it go.

Over time, this practice, perhaps, will serve to create larger openings to Self. It is no more than a dis-identification practice, but it shifts its emphasis to the self-identification end. It invites the space, between all identifications to grow. Perhaps, in our contemplation, the psychological functions will each release more easily, more quickly and the empty space between the steps of the practice will be longer. Perhaps this is, as Assagioli describes it, the "state of perfect repose, an inner silence, taking the form of pure consciousness." (1991, p. 36) Perhaps one day, the breath and the silence, the pure consciousness, will be all there is…

and then the doorbell will ring.

With a smile, we will welcome our personality back, knowing that it has remembered where the car keys are, knows where the cheque book is, has already planned dinner. Self, manifesting in your unique personality moves from the cushion and gladly welcomes the guest who rings the bell.

References

Assagioli, R, *Psychosynthesis*, Hobbs, Dorman & Co., 1965

Assagioli, R, *Transpersonal Development*, HarperCollins Publishers, 1991

Assagioli, R, 'Psychosynthesis', *Synthesis Center Press*, 2000 (12th printing)

Assagioli, R., 'The Act of Will', *Synthesis Center Press*, 2010

Brown, MY, *Unfolding Self: The Practice of Psychosynthesis*, Helios Press, 2004

Firmin, J, and Gila, A, 'Psychosynthesis: A Psychology of the Spirit' in *Transpersonal and Humanistic Psychology*, SUNY Series, 2002

Seng-Ts'an, *Hsin Hsin Ming*, Verses on the Faith-Mind, Clarke, RB (trans.), White Pines Press, 2001

Danté and the Transformation of Despair

Group Relations in Psychosynthesis and their Role in Creating Hellish States of Mind or Blissful Collaborations

Jarlath F. Benson

Danté Alighieri is the great poet of despair and bliss who plumbed the very depths and heights of human experience. He describes the deliverance of the human Soul from a spiritually dead and self-centred life and offers a model for transforming Despair into Dialogue and Hope which is particularly relevant for the modern psychosynthesis group worker.

Danté was born in 1265 and was a renowned poet who lived in Florence and was involved in the politics and government of the city until his party was deposed by a rival faction and he was exiled. He never returned to Florence. This was an enormous source of pain to him for the rest of his life and was a huge motivating factor in his writing the classic poem *The Divine Comedy* (Musa, 1995, from which all quotations from the poem in this paper are taken). *The Divine Comedy* has continuously inspired all generations since because of its central idea that human life is a pilgrimage inspired by love – an odyssey from error to truth, from darkness to light, from isolation and alienation to complete association and communion.

It is made up of three sections: Hell, known as the Inferno, is inhabited by those who have been separated from the social body and are alienated and isolated; Purgatory is an harmonious society in which everyone accepts responsibility for their actions, behaves socially and deplores damage to others; in Paradiso the human is pure spirit devoid of selfishness and constitutes the ideal society.

Retribution is the keynote of the Inferno. Hope is the promise of the Purgatorio. Fellowship and love is the essential nature of the Paradiso. Danté sets out plainly to illustrate the pitfalls and consequences of moral degeneracy as a consequence of pathological narcissism and lack of relationship; he indicates the steps of moral purification and refinement of consciousness through creating mutual and ethical group relations and he gives a clear vision of the underlying reality of human life.

Although the Divine Comedy appears to be a model of spiritual development set within a medieval Christian context it is also a profound meditation on the deepest and enduring realities underpinning human groups. Danté asserts that humans are essentially relational beings and insists that the individual personal and social are inextricably interconnected. We are each responsible for the welfare and quality of life of our fellows and they for us. Human beings in order to be human beings cannot exist outside a group or community and must contribute actively to it. Civic action and group engagement are therefore some of the highest forms of moral or immoral activity.

Danté's expressed aim is to move the human from a state of misery to a state of happiness and he is clear that his poem is a most practical guide emphasising the vital importance of mutual relations and collaborative sharing. This contrasts with the aim of Freud who declared that the purpose of Psychoanalysis was to help men move from "neurotic misery to common human unhappiness."

Central to the poem is the importance of corrective emotional experience painfully gained as a result of the process of learning and teaching fundamental truths. The Commedia is a celebration of learning and acquiring knowledge and provides profound insight into the growth of the human mind. Unwilling to acquire right knowledge the minds of the spirits in hell are permanently clouded – in Purgatory the spirits are gradually enlightened and in Paradiso the spirits have reached complete happiness because they share in total knowledge with the Omniscient organising principle which for Danté is God.

Right knowledge for Danté is about the reality of and search for human and cosmic interconnectedness and the pursuit of the means of transformation of that regressive narcissism which results in self-idolatry and the extinction of civilised relations. Underpinning this vision is Danté's insistence on the centrality of Free Will and moral responsibility on the part of the human. No psychic determinist – Danté is unambiguous; the individual must hold himself responsible for his actions and the words he utters and such action must be deliberate and graded if it is not to distance us from the love of God and from each other.

The Structure and Narrative of the Divine Comedy

The Commedia is an immense and complex creation – more than 14 thousand lines long and any introduction to it must be a humble endeavour providing the reader with a few insights to undertake the journey Danté lays before us. The dramatic action of the poem describes Danté's exploration and journey through an immense poetic universe into which we are invited as fellow travellers. The topography of this universe is divided into three regions. Hell is a triangular shaped hole in the earth created when Lucifer, the most brilliant of the angels, was cast out of Heaven after his rebellion and physically plunged into matter. From a modern psychological perspective it corresponds to the deep unconscious or shadow aspect of the human. Danté moves down into the centre of the earth to the Satanic core of Hell under the guidance of the wise Virgil, investigating various discrete regions where specific modes of sinfulness are punished in symbolically apt ways. The general movement downward reflects an increasing degree of severity and pathology. The gates of Hell are marked by those infamous lines: "Abandon every hope All you who enter" (1995, Canto III, Line 9).

The deeper the pilgrim goes, the more he – and we – learn about the psychology of sin and the structure of the human shadow. By the time this part of the journey ends, Danté is sufficiently aware of the nature of evil – that evil is a frozen and embittered human heart and a refusal to relate with or consider others – to begin the purgative process that leads ultimately to God and right relationships.

The material displaced by Lucifer's fall to earth is pushed out on the other side of our planet as a mountain called Purgatory that Danté painfully ascends in the poem. Whereas Inferno deals with the effects of narcissistic relationships, Purgatorio deals with the causes of narcissistic relationships and insists that the only way of transforming self-centredness is through contrition and the recognition that one must learn new ways of relating to oneself and others. This requires self-examination and the actual telling and revealing of one's shadow to others. In group therapy this is the most difficult of steps and is often experienced as a humiliation but is in fact restorative because it is an attempt at making restitution for what has been lost through previous self-indulgence and self-absorption by emphasising a participatory and other-centred attitude to life. As in group psychotherapy Danté gives us a picture in Purgatorio of souls learning to work together to make reconnection and provides a precise model which includes dream analysis, cultivating the inner life of imagination, fostering an aesthetic sensibility and specific guides to collaborative relations.

The third realm is Paradiso in which the techniques for higher states of consciousness and creative collaboration are elaborated. Mutual mirroring, right vision and loving relations are central to the transformation of narcissistic preoccupations and are continual refrains and motifs beautifully described in the Commedia:

The more souls there are above who are in love
The more there are worth loving: love grows more
Each soul a mirror mutually mirroring.
(Purgatorio, Canto XV, Lines 73-5)

So it is clear that Souls who see properly love more and make themselves thereby better 'reflectors' of God's love. (Paradiso, Canto XIV, Lines 33-60.) One who sees the world properly will be filled with love for God and other people; one who is not imbued with such love will demonstrate that he or she has not properly seen the world and mistakenly makes their own self the world centre. Getting the vision 'right', seeing the world as it really is increases the capacity to love mutually and relate reciprocally. Perhaps we can come close to a perception of Danté's Paradiso by recalling De Maré's concept of Koinonia applied to large groups which he defines as "spiritual-cum-human participation in which people can speak, hear and see, and think freely, a form of togetherness and amity that brings a pooling of resources" (de Maré et al, 1991, p. 2).

The poem begins with Danté lost in a famous allegorical landscape.

Midway along the journey of our life I woke to find myself in a dark wood
For I had wandered off from the straight path.
How hard it is to tell what it was like
This wood of wilderness, savage and stubborn
The very thought of it brings back all my old fears.
A bitter place! Death could scarce be bitterer
But if I would show the good that came of it I must talk about things other than the good.
(Canto 1, Lines 1-9)

The symbolic and psychological implications of the scene are clear. Danté realises he is in a profound existential crisis and must face circumstances and creatures who represent threats to his soul's survival if he is to recover the knowledge of how to live creatively and hopefully. The Dark Wood is the experience of a Hardenss of Heart in which a pathological narcissism has so possessed the soul as to render it incapable of turning to God or knowing which way to turn (cf. Sayers, 1949, p. 73). This mention of sin and evil may make you uneasy but it is important to remember that Danté is a medieval Christian writer whose theology does not undermine the profound psychological value of his insights into the human condition. We can easily reframe sin and evil as a regressive narcissism that hardens and freezes the heart and makes all others objects with no value at all and eventually extinguishes civil relations.

Danté beholds the Mountain of Purgation and Repentance. It can be ascended from 'the right road' but not from the Dark Wood because there the Soul's cherished aims have become externalised and appear to it as demons or beasts with a will and power of their own, blocking all progress. Once lost in the Dark Wood a person can only escape by descending within the self so as to see sin not as an external obstacle but as the perverted will to chaos and death within the human. But Danté offers us – the living souls – the remedial possibility of journeying on our behalf through the hellish state and revealing for our self-knowledge the nature of impenitent sin and all its evil potentialities.

As Danté journeys through hell, purgatory and paradise, therefore, he is also going through states of personal and human potential, and we accompany him on this pilgrimage from darkness to light, from ignorance to wisdom. He has three guides through the otherworld: Virgil guides Danté from the dark wood, through Inferno, up Mount Purgatory to the Earthly Paradise. Virgil is the embodiment of human reason – an image of a masculine analytic mentality – that we can reframe as a traditional model of psychotherapy. This can only go so far and must give way to Beatrice who is an incarnation of a feminine intuitive wisdom mind. In psychosynthesis terms Beatrice might represent the maternal container and I-Self function of individual and group psychotherapy.

Beatrice was for Danté an actual woman in her own right whom he deeply loved but she also represented for him an image of nobility, of virtue, of the redeemed life and in some sense an experience of *Almighty God* Himself who manifests through her. Beatrice guides Danté from the Earthly Paradise, up through the various circles of heaven; and St. Bernard of Clairvaux takes over in the final stages leading Danté into the permanent presence of God and the ideal society. Danté's overall theme is that *Love pervades the universe* and that we human beings either find harmony in that love or by opposing God's love, damage the creation, ourselves and the others around us.

Danté powerfully asserts that the love between two humans is one of the most powerful inducements to come alive to the love of God. The individual who loves narcissistically – *love of an earthly object for its own sake rather than seeing it as a manifestation of the divine* – removes himself further from Charity which is the source and goal, the true 'cosmic force of generation'. Such a Lover lacks the vision and reason which would instruct and illuminate him both to the personal reality of the beloved and the realisation that the beloved is a vessel for the manifestation of Divine Love.

Beatrice is the woman who initially draws Danté into and onto the path that leads towards Universal Love. This path consists of a series of graded and ordered loves and relationships spread over the entire universe but it starts for Danté with the love for a woman providing the entry point for a deep encounter with Divine Love. Danté's love for Beatrice is ennobling and spiritual and it is passionate and in his view this personal passion fits in with God's universal scheme of redemption and correct relationship.

Love then is the generative force in the universe as Danté recounts in canto17 of the Purgatorio:

Neither creator nor his creatures ever, My son, lacked love. There are as you well know, Two kinds: the natural love, the rational.

Natural love may never be at fault; The other may be: by choosing the wrong goal, By insufficient or excessive zeal.

While it is fixed on the Eternal Good, And observes temperance loving worldly goods, It cannot be the cause of sinful joys;

But when it turns towards evil or pursues Some good with not enough or too much zeal The creature turns on his Creator then.

So you can understand how love must be The seeds of every virtue growing in you, And every deed that merits punishment.

(Canto XVII, Lines 91-105)

Danté is very clear: the Creator and every creature is moved by love but this supreme love, which is no other than the love of God, may err by an act of will or choice and being so misdirected may become perverse and evil. In canto 16 Danté explains his understanding of the relation of human will to Divine Will:

You men on earth attribute everything To the sphere's influence alone as if With some predestined plan they moved all things.

If this were true, then our Free Will would be Annihilated: it would not be just To render bliss for good or pain for evil.
The spheres initiate your tendencies: Not all of them – but even if they did, You have the light that shows you right from wrong.
And your Free will, which, though it may grow faint In its first struggles with the heavens, can still Surmount all obstacles if nurtured well.
You are free subjects of a greater power, A nobler nature that creates your mind And over this the spheres have no control.
(Purgatorio, Canto XVI, Lines 67-81)

And again in Canto XVIII:
You have the innate faculty of reason
Which should defend the threshold of consent.
This is the principle on which is based The judgement of your merit – according as It winnows out the good love from the bad.
Those men who with their reason probed the depths Perceived this liberty in man Thereby bequeathing ethics to the world.
Let us assume that every love that burns In you arises through necessity; You still have the power to restrain such love.
This noble Beatrice knows As Freedom of the Will: remember that If ever she should mention it to you.
(Lines 62-75)

So it is clear: human beings are fundamentally motivated by love. But an individual or group can love too much; can love too little or love the wrong thing. The twin towers bombers are lovers. The paedophile is a lover. Hitler was a lover. But the path of love requires reason and discrimination and the careful and educated exercise of one's free will and choice because on the journey of the soul the object of one's love is *not just the thing in itself but also the love of God who is manifesting and sacramentalising the object.*

Thus the informing and compelling wellspring of the Divine Comedy is Love – not a love restricted to the idealisation of one passion but the articulation of a force that impels every creature to obey the highest dictates of its nature. Danté's simple but profound message is that love permeates the universe and human beings, through the exercise of reason and will, either cooperate with or turn away from love and in so doing are elevated to the best of themselves or are degraded to the worst of themselves.

In this sense Danté's towering poem is a medieval draft of a complete psychosynthesis as Roberto Assagioli averred. Psychosynthesis asserts the importance of right relations and is a central part of the training in the Institute of Psychosynthesis in London. The practice of right group relations offers the alienated and self-absorbed individual a second chance – an opportunity to engage in ordered and graduated mutual and loving relationships in which desire can be re-educated and appropriately re-directed. The sterile isolation and self-congratulatory monologues of Inferno are gradually and with the assistance of a wise guide transmuted into the conversations and mutual ambitions of a developing community so characteristic of Purgatorio. And finally the loving relations of Paradiso mirror a delight and a concern with persons and existences other than ourselves that at times evokes and catalyses experiences of exaltation and transcendence.

The pure spirituality, radiant charity and ineffable tenderness of Danté's vision ensure that his text remains a classic that never belongs to the past but always to the present. It carries a permanent message of psychosynthesis group relations and significance for all generations and still makes a direct and universal appeal to the heart and the conscience after 700 years.

References

Benson, JF, *Working More Creatively With Groups*, Routledge, 2001

De Maré, P, Piper, R and Thompson. S, *Koinonia: From Hate through Dialogue to Culture in the Large Group*, Karnac Books, 1991

Musa, M, *The Portable Danté*, Viking Portable Library, Pelican Books, 1995

Sayers, DL, *The Divine Comedy,* Cantica I Hell, Penguin Classics, 1949

Website Links: http://en.wikipedia.org/wiki/Divine_Comedy

The Deep River Within

Abby Seixas

Abby Seixas's book *Finding the Deep River Within: A Woman's Guide to Recovering Balance and Meaning in Everyday Life*, published by Jossey-Bass, an imprint of Wiley & Sons in 2006, explores how we can connect to a deeper sense of self in order to bring greater meaning and well-being to our lives. In this chapter, reproduced with the kind permission of the author and publisher, Abby introduces the concept of the 'Deep River' and provides a simple exercise to help us tap into this resource, draw nourishment from it and return to life 'at the surface' with renewed perspective and vitality.

In the face of 'too much' we gradually become dry, our hearts get tired, our energies become spare, and a mysterious longing for – we almost never have a name for it other than 'a something' – rises up in us more and more… (Clarissa Pinkola Estés, 1992)

When we get the urge to simplify and slow down, most of us tend to think, "I just need to get more organized". Although time management might be helpful, it can also be one of those 'solutions' that is part of the problem: we manage our time better so that we can more efficiently pack more activity into our already overpacked schedules.

My view, and the approach of this book, is that we need to look in an entirely different, sometimes unfamiliar, direction for a solution to the sense of overwhelm. To regain our balance and find meaning and satisfaction in how we live, we need to 'drop down' and look underneath the perpetual-motion busyness of our daily lives.

From Surface to Depth

When I speak of looking underneath or dropping down, I am talking about moving from a more outward focus at the surface of our lives, to a more inward focus deep within ourselves. The diagram later in this chapter illustrates this movement. We can move from surface to depth, or outer to inner, because we all have a place of depth within us, whether or not we are aware of it at any given time. This place of depth might be thought of as the spiritual dimension within us. There are many names for this inner realm, and probably as many different experiences of it as there are people. Some describe it as 'going home', for some it is the place for contact with the 'still small voice' within; others say it is where they go in themselves to reconnect with God, with meaning, or with a 'bigger picture' sense of their life; or for spiritual renewal, or for creative inspiration. I often have the image when I drop down or go inside, of an underground river that is always there, always flowing through me, from a source beyond me, carrying deeply nourishing, life-giving qualities. After I first saw the Deep River in my mind's eye, I discovered that it is not my image alone. Jungian analyst and author Clarissa Estés writes of the *rio abajo rio*, "the river beneath the river, which flows and flows into our lives" (Estés 1992, p. 298). May Sarton (1973, p. 145) writes of the "deep still water" where dreams and images live. When Jessie, the main character in Sue Monk Kidd's *The Mermaid Chair*, longed for a more authentic, satisfying life, she described the feeling that "there had to be some other life beneath the one I had, like an underground river or something, and that I would die if I didn't dig down to it" (2005, p. 309).

My name for this place of depth is the Deep River within. We all have this dimension within us, but we differ in what we find there as well as how we experience it. Janine, a woman in one of my groups, describes her experience in this straightforward way: "When I go there, time slows down, I get clarity, and the self-talk tape shuts off." Another group member refers to the Psalm celebrating "the secret place of the Most High" to help her orient toward the Deep River realm. She says, "I tend to think of the Deep River as the place where the noise stops and a sense of peace and stillness finally takes over. It's the place where I *feel* rather than *think* my true nature." Another woman describes it as "where I disconnect from the chatter so that I can connect to what is real for me, what makes my heart sing, what pains me, and what is important to me."

Of course, the Deep River is not a physical destination. A favourite corner of the living room or an especially beautiful natural setting might be *conducive* to tapping into the Deep River realm, but the Deep River is a state of consciousness rather than an actual place.

Marie, a graphic designer, found that drawing brought her to the Deep River within. "When I am drawing and relaxed it feels like I am in a tunnel where there are no distractions around me…I am not aware of my body at all or anyone or anything for that matter. My sense of time is suspended and I am deeply concentrated. I trust that my hand 'knows' and that I need to get out of the way to allow it to just move and feel and not direct it. This is not easy to do because my mind and judgment often get in the way. But when it does work, it is a very relaxed and deeply satisfying state."

Deep River Qualities

While everyone's experience of this Deep River state is different, certain qualities are often described. For example:

- Peace, calm
- Silence, stillness
- Aliveness, vitality
- Gratitude, grace
- Clarity, perspective
- Creativity, inspiration
- Joy, contentment
- Fluidity, ease
- Trusting, letting go
- Tenderness, love
- Groundedness, solidity
- Wholeness, sense of self
- Universality, sense of connection to others
- Compassion – for one's own and others' suffering

This is not a comprehensive list. One or more of these qualities, or perhaps something not listed, might describe your experience of contact with the Deep River realm. Don't be surprised if this contact has a bittersweet quality – our deepest experiences often contain a poignant mixture of light and dark, joy and sorrow. The exercise at the end of this chapter is designed to take you to your own experience of what I am describing here, whatever its particular qualities are for you.

In Deep River experiences, one's sense of time is almost always altered. Janine says that time slows down, and Marie says that her sense of time is suspended. Another woman says that time "opens up", while another says, "I feel when I am in this place that I have all the time in the world." These comments reflect the reality that our sense of time is subjective and malleable. When we are totally absorbed in something – a creative endeavour or a conversation with a friend – what seemed like a half hour can actually turn out to be two or three. In the Deep River realm, time is not experienced as linear, constraining and stressful the way it often is in the rest of our lives. Rather, we have a sense of timelessness, or spaciousness. Time, or lack of it, ceases to be the enemy. That is why we need to look toward the Deep River within to find balance in our harried lives: perhaps it actually isn't more time that we need, but a different way of experiencing the time we have.

The Value of the Deep River

Some of you reading this chapter may recognize the Deep River realm as familiar territory. Others may be wondering "What is this for *me*?" Or, "Even if I assume I have a place of depth within me, how do I find it?" Having questions like these does *not* mean something is wrong with you. The prevailing culture neither teaches us about nor values this inner realm, much less shows us how to gain access to it. So, most of us need support for making contact with the Deep River within, but first we must understand *why* this contact is important.

Clarissa Estés describes what happens when we are cut off from our inner selves using the archetypal story, told in many northern countries throughout the world, of the seal woman. The water is the seal woman's home, what we might call her place of depth. Although she belongs to the sea, and lives beneath the water as a seal, by night she can take human form. One night, she and her seal-sisters shed their pelts and dance naked atop a rock by the sea. A lonely man comes upon them and steals the seal woman's pelt before she can put it back on and slip back into the sea, pleading with her to be his wife. Estés says of the pelt, "[it] is not so much an article as the representation of a feeling state and a state of being – one that is cohesive, soulful, and of the wildish female nature. When a woman is in this state, she feels entirely in and of herself..." (*ibid*, p. 265). And being without the pelt "causes a woman to pursue what she thinks she should do, rather than what she truly wishes" (*ibid*, p. 269).

The seal woman agrees to remain with the lonely man, but when she stays too long on land, away from the depths, without her pelt, she begins to dry out. Her skin cracks, her hair thins, she begins to limp, and her eyes lose their moisture. This dried-out state, "peeling, limping, losing juice, going blind" is a good metaphorical description of what happens when we have no access to our own depths. Our lives seem flat, dry and empty, even if they are full of activity, people and things. We feel as if we are going through the motions of life, but not really living.

The seal woman's over-long stay on land points to another effect of being cut off from our deeper nature: we are more prone to physical symptoms of stress, to addictive behaviour, to conflict and disconnection in our relationships, to less satisfaction in our work, and in our lives. We need to be able to find our way back to our water-home for replenishment and renewal. In the story, when the seal woman finally breaks free from the man, reclaims her pelt and returns to the sea, the shine returns to her hair and eyes, her sight is restored, her body becomes plump and full and strong again. Access to the deeper realms within us gives back us our 'juice', our vital energy and resilience. We return to our true selves, or in Estés' language, we return to home and to being wholly in our skins, which in turn can help us relate more fully and openly to others and to the activities we engage in. We find a sense of connection to something larger than our own individual concerns, and a sense of meaning that makes what we do with our time feel worthwhile.

Janet, a young mother of two, experienced the value of this contact when she began to take time each day to, in her words, "find my deeper self", and to practice staying in touch with her depth in the midst of her daily interactions. She said, "If I approach relationships from that deeper place instead of the more superficial place, I'm more 'responsible' not responsible in the sense of taking charge, but more responsible in the sense of able-to-respond." As an example, she described a typical afternoon when her son was sitting in the next room doing some homework. "I was rushing around the kitchen like a chicken with its head cut off, cleaning, with a sense of urgency. My son asked me a question; he wanted my attention. My tendency is to say, "When I'm done", and continue with a sense of urgency. So at first I said "in a little while", and then I had an awareness, because I'm practicing this, that I was very revved up. I noticed it in my body, all this tension and unnecessary movement, and I made an effort to quiet my body. Then my mind got more quiet, and I said, "Yeah, I'll be right there. I can do this a little later." I went in with a sense of calm and quiet, and I was able to really connect with him in a way that was relaxing and fulfilling for both of us. I know that's what he wanted – to connect with me, with *me*, not that person who was cleaning counters with urgency. As an afterthought, she said, "By the way, there was no urgency, really. It was just a *sense* of urgency, the sense that nothing will ever be done, the sense of *what is going to happen if I stop now, for 15 minutes, when I have to finish cleaning the kitchen, put in a load of laundry...blah, blah, blah.* That's the so-called urgency!"

After she described her experience, Janet said, "It's even better because when I went back to cleaning the counters, I could remember why I was doing it. I remembered what all this is for...it's for the family." As she said this, Janet began to tear up. In describing this interaction, she seemed to recognise what truly mattered to her. She said, "It's really about coming from that place of loving, and the doing gets in the way of the loving, but we just don't see that most of the time. And all of the doing is *because* of the loving, but it gets in the way." Then she added, "There's so much tenderness in that deep place, that we don't have access to so much of the time."

Visualising the Deep River

Janet's experience speaks to the effect that 'dropping down' can have on life 'at the surface. Of course sometimes urgency is real and we can't take time to sit down and talk with our children. But often, especially in a cultural context that values speed and doing, we, like Janet, stay at the surface of our lives, keeping busy with a false sense of urgency, and missing opportunities to engage in fulfilling ways with those we love, or with ourselves, or even with a mundane task such as cleaning the counter.

So, how do we gain access to and draw on the inner resources that bring deep nourishment or 'juice' as Estés puts it, to our ordinary lives? I developed the diagram over the page over many years of working with women to help them visualize both the process and the essential tools necessary to open up access to the Deep River. As I've said before, touching the depth within us is not something we can simply add to the To-Do list or squeeze in as we go from one errand to another. The Deep River realm may unexpectedly break through life's routines, but more often we have to exert conscious effort to create the conditions that open us to this dimension. There may be some cultures in which people don't have to work to drop down and touch the Deep River, but in our culture of speed, interruption and distraction, without conscious effort we will remain at the surface.

Women in my groups have used the diagram as a reminder that it is possible to slow down and connect with what matters. They keep a copy of it in their datebooks, post it next to their computers, tape it to their refrigerators and dashboards. One group member says, "I have a copy of the diagram taped to a wall along with some favourite sayings, near where I meditate. I put it there because I love the concept of 'dropping down' that's embodied in it, and because it's a clear reminder of what it is I'm working on".

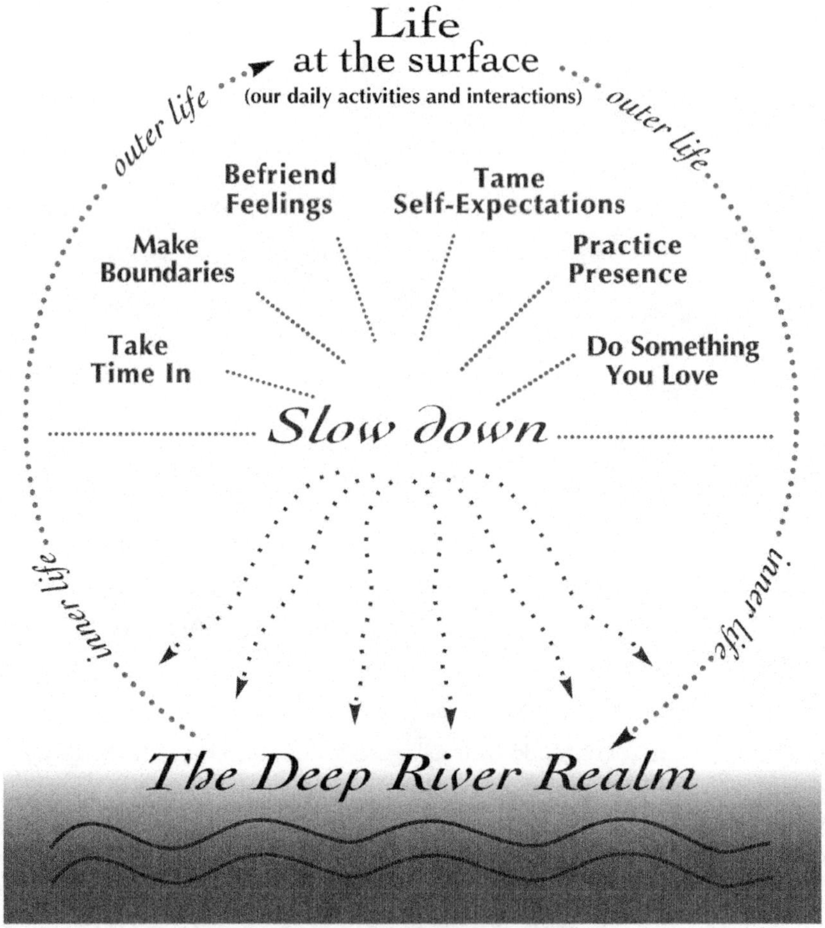

The Deep River Process
From *Finding the Deep River Within: A Woman's Guide to Recovering Balance and Meaning in Everyday Life* by Abby Seixas (Jossey-Bass. 2006)
www.deepriverwithin.com
© 2006 Deep River Seminars

The Key: Slowing Down

In the centre of the diagram, in bold italic letters, are the words, "SLOW DOWN". At least in 21st century North America, this is the most fundamental prerequisite for receiving nourishment from the Deep River within. To see the importance of slowing down, consider this brief exercise:

Imagine a beautiful summer garden in full bloom on a sunny day, with all the colours and scents, shapes and textures of a variety of flowers and shrubs. Take a moment right now to picture this garden, however you see it in your mind's eye. Imagine wandering through it on a winding path, perhaps stopping now and gazing at whatever flowers you are drawn to. Notice the colours and shapes of the flowers you are looking at. Imagine you can breathe in the colours and breathe in the beauty you see, just as you might be breathing in the scent. Notice what happens in your body as you imagine inhaling this beauty.

Now, imagine you are driving in a car at 60 miles an hour. Off to your right is a beautiful summer garden in full bloom on a sunny day. Oops...it's gone by. Did you catch it? We might notice a blur of colour before it's gone, and we might tell others that we saw a beautiful garden while we were driving, but there is simply no way we can truly take in the garden's beauty, let it touch us and be nourished by it, while speeding by at 60 miles an hour.

Despite what our faster-is-better culture may tell us, we *do* need to slow down if we want to open up access to the Deep River within. There is no question that this can be difficult; a habitually fast pace has its own momentum that is hard to break. If we're used to living in overdrive, slowing down may become hard to tolerate; we may feel uncomfortable, unproductive, bored, restless, at a slower pace. If it's uncomfortable, we may not stop until we encounter life events that *throw* us off the treadmill, forcing us to slow down at least temporarily, which can result in opening us up to depth.

For Louise, a mother of two who worked full-time, the event that shifted her own life dramatically happened to someone she was close to. Louise had worked hard for fifteen years at a job in sales and marketing which, she said, "sucked the life right out of me". Looking back at her life then, Louise described it as "totally externally-focused, driven, and very out of control". During that time, one of Louise's friends was in a very severe car accident. It was unclear whether she would survive. During one of the first nights that her friend was in the hospital, Louise slept only intermittently, thinking and dreaming about her and her family for what seemed like most of the night. She said, "Toward morning, just as I was awakening – I was no longer sleeping but I really was not awake either – I had this thought about my friend: 'Even if her life is over now, she can *know* that she has done a great job as a mother'. Then all of a sudden I applied that thought to myself, and I remember the clutching feeling in my chest. It was a visceral reaction as I thought: 'If I were to die tomorrow, that couldn't be said about me'". She saw that she had been so distracted by her job that she wasn't 'living her values', which to her meant putting her children first. The incongruity between what she believed in and how she was living was so stark and jolting to her in that moment that she had to act. "I gave my notice to a job that I'd had for fifteen years, I didn't go for options, I didn't think about how else I might resolve this. It was completely: I've got to stop this freight train, and get off".

The next several months were hard in a different way for Louise. She was at home and spending much more time with her children, but she still felt driven and could not settle down. "I was sewing pillow-covers with a vengeance! I felt enormous stress, but now most of it was self-generated." Eventually, in an effort to address the stress she was feeling both physically and emotionally, Louise attended a weekend retreat that included some guided visualisation. At first, she had trouble focusing her attention inwardly, but on one of the 'inner journeys', she found herself able to truly go inside, and her inner world opened up. She went in her mind's eye back to her childhood home, and re-contacted a deep sense of loneliness that had been with her often as a child. She realised that in her adult life, the 'freight train' energy that caused her so much stress was fuelled in part by trying to avoid the old feeling of discomfort with quiet aloneness from her childhood. This awareness helped her with the changes she wanted to make. Later she said, "I had lived my life for so long in an outer fashion, and I was so out of synch and so screwed up. I had some sense that I needed to look inside, but it was so hard. I didn't know how to do it".

Her weekend retreat was the beginning of an inner exploration that led Louise to one of my groups, among other things, and eventually, as her children got older, to an entirely new career that connects back to that early-morning moment that affected her so profoundly: she teaches, trains and writes about parenting skills. "What I'm doing now uses all of who I am: my professional experience, my skill, my education. And it's married to my passion. So it's very powerful for me. And now, because what I'm doing is inner-driven, there's an energy and an authenticity about it that keeps me going."

Sadly, the norms of our non-stop way of life mean that one of the most frequently travelled paths to the Deep River is through crisis, such as serious illness, death of a loved one, divorce, or some other major loss. Whether they happen to ourselves or, like Louise, to someone close to us, such events stop us in our tracks, prompting us to look inward. The Deep River process is based on the contention that we don't have to wait until we are in shock or in terrible pain to begin to find our way to the depth within. We can intentionally, consciously create conditions that invite the Deep River to flow into our lives.

Dropping Down and Returning to the Surface

Encircling the diagram are two arrows representing the movement that we are seeking to create in our day-to-day living, from surface to depth, and back to the surface again. The goal of this book is not to encourage retreating to a cave or monastery to live out our days in silence. Rather, the goal is to establish a consistent rhythm within our daily routine that allows us to tap into the Deep River, draw nourishment from it, and return to life "at the surface" with renewed perspective and vitality, remembering what really matters to us. In this way, what we do in our outer lives (our daily activities and interactions) is informed by our inner lives and gives expression to the qualities of the Deep River realm.

As I write this, it's winter in New England. Last week nature provided a region-wide enforced slow-down in the form of a blizzard. In the days after the storm, several of my clients described having spent their 'snow day' at a slower pace, taking time off, doing things they ordinarily would not have taken time for. My own sense of the day was one of unburdened spaciousness, as if the yoke of time had temporarily lifted itself off of me and everyone around me. Aside from shovelling snow, the weather forced a kind of Sabbath, a day of rest. The cycle of activity/rest/and return is crucial to being able to maintain balance and energy in our lives, and yet, short of a blizzard or another motion-stopping event, we override and push past the "rest" part of the cycle again and again. The poet May Sarton writes of this need for rest and the tendency to override it in her *Journal of A Solitude*: "A strange empty day. I did not feel well; lay around, looked at daffodils against the white walls…I always forget how important the empty days are, how important it may be sometimes not to expect to produce anything, even a few lines in a journal. I am still pursued by a neurosis about work inherited from my father. A day where one has not pushed oneself to the limit seems a damaged damaging day, a sinful day. Not so! The most valuable thing we can do for the psyche, occasionally, is to let it rest, wander, live in the changing light of a room, not try to be or do anything whatever. Tonight I do feel in a state of grace, limbered up, less strained" (*ibid*, p. 89).

Sarton is describing the renewing effect of stepping out of the habitual mode of produce-produce-produce, and allowing one's whole being to pause. I want to highlight the importance of the cycle that the arrows in the diagram represent. That cycle, of activity/dropping down/and return, is the antithesis of what has been so aptly named our 24/7 way of life.

The Practices

Above the words 'Slow down' on the diagram are six radiating lines, each with the name of one of the six essential tools or practices to open up access to the Deep River realm. These tools have a reciprocal relationship to slowing down. That is, slowing down makes it easier to do each practice, and when we do each practice, it helps us to slow down. In brief, the six essential practices are:

1 *Take time-in*: Learn to gather energy and find balance by taking uninterrupted alone-time to drop below the surface of daily activity.

2 *Befriend feelings*: Learn to accept and make friends with uncomfortable feelings that you may be trying to avoid by keeping busy.
3 *Make boundaries*: Learn the primary skill for heading off the feeling of being overwhelmed: how to say 'no'.
4 *Tame self-expectations*: Learn to lighten up and take the self-critical voice of perfectionism less seriously.
5 *Practice presence*: Learn to address *mental* busyness, through cultivating mindfulness of the present moment.
6 *Do something you love*: Learn to create time to experience the renewing power of doing something simply for the enjoyment of doing it.

As the arrows in the lower half of the diagram indicate, each of these practices, in combination with slowing down, is a potential doorway to the Deep River dimension. In addition, there are three preliminary practices designed to help you get started: *Recognise the Power of the Culture, Get Support,* and *Keep a Journal.* Should you choose to learn more about the three preliminary and six core practices of the Deep River process, you will begin to see how each practice on its own can be beneficial, as well as how all of them fit together. In the meantime, a good place to start is with an exercise to connect with your own experience of the Deep River realm.

Exercise: Re-Living a Deep River Experience

Before we move on to the specific practices for connecting with the Deep River within, I encourage you to take a few moments to do a guided visualisation exercise that will help you experience what we have been talking about. I have found that we all have some experience of the Deep River realm, even if we haven't touched into it for weeks, months or years. This exercise helps you remember one of these times, and reconnect with the body sensations, feelings and thoughts that accompany it. Re-living a positive experience of your inner nature can provide motivation to invite more contact with this dimension in your daily life. Reconnecting with your experience of the Deep River is important, too, because *experience* is the most valuable of all 'tools' for slowing down, simplifying, and reclaiming your life.

To get the most from the exercise, find a place and time when you will be undisturbed. You won't need a lot of time – even ten minutes of uninterrupted time is enough. Read through the exercise first. The words are meant to guide you toward an inner experience that is beyond words. They are only guidelines – you don't have to follow them exactly. After you have read through the exercise, do it at your own pace.

You can also have a friend read the exercise to you slowly, with some pauses to allow you to contact your experience. Take time to make some notes of your own before you reciprocate and guide your friend through the exercise.

Close your eyes. Sit comfortably in a chair and consciously relax your body. Imagine your muscles loosening and let go of any tension you may be holding in them. Take a few moments to focus your attention on your breathing; allow the rhythm of your breath to quiet you and help focus your attention inside yourself.

Now, think of a time when you may have 'touched the Deep River'. This may have been a time when you felt very energized or very calmed by being in nature, or felt a sense of wonder at the natural world; or it may have been an experience of being awed by something beautiful, or an experience of communion with another person, or with God; or just a sense of a loving presence, some force larger than yourself that you were part of. It may have been an experience of great joy, or love, or gratitude for simply being alive. It may have been a time when you experienced a very clear insight about something troubling you or about how life works or the meaning of your life. Or a time when you felt somehow very fully yourself, very whole, fully alive.

Take your time to allow a memory of this experience to present itself. There is no one 'right' experience. It can be something that happened very recently, or all the way back in your childhood. It can be an experience you had during an ordinary everyday activity, like washing the dishes, or during an important life event, like giving birth.

When you think of a time when you had this heightened awareness, make it as vivid as possible in your imagination. Allow yourself to re-live it as fully as you can. What sensations do you notice in your body? Let yourself re-experience any sensations that accompanied the experience, including sights, sounds, smells. Let yourself experience the feelings you felt, the thoughts you had. How did you experience the people around you, the world around you?

Take all the time you need to re-live this experience. When you have a good sense of it, see if you can name for yourself the quality (or qualities) at the heart of this experience. Is it peace, or joy, gratitude, clarity, wonder, acceptance, silence, caring, wholeness… what is it for you?

Take your time, and when you are ready, you can gently open your eyes, and if you wish, take some notes.

Touching in to your own experience of the Deep River realm is the first step toward allowing more of its restorative waters flow into your everyday life. I wish you well on the journey!

References

Estés, CP, *Women Who Run With the Wolves*, Ballantine Books, 1992

Kidd, SM, *The Mermaid Chair*, Viking, 2005

Sarton, M, *Journal of a Solitude*, WW Norton & Co., 1973

Seixas, A, *Finding the Deep River Within: A Woman's Guide to Recovering Balance and Meaning in Everyday Life*, Jossey-Bass, an imprint of Wiley & Sons, 2006

Archetypal Psychosynthesis or the Psychology of Unity: A New Look at the 'Egg Diagram'

Dr Kristina Brode

We are approaching the level of an archetypal consciousness.
(Stanislav Grof, 2011)

My Experiences with the Psychosynthesis Egg Diagram

I love the Egg Diagram. And people love to be taught this model. I see myself at a bedside in the hospital introducing myself and my work there to the cancer patient waiting to have surgery the next day. One of my first sentences is: "I work with psychosynthesis to reach our goals here: to minimize your distress, let you find more inner peace and remind you of the strength that you have proved so often in your life".

The question that always comes back is: 'Never heard of this, what is psychosynthesis?'

With my writing pad on my knees I draw the Egg, with its dotted lines and boundaries, and describe our inner life of often conflicting subpersonalities (who does not know "the two souls in his chest"), their dependency and connectedness. I explain how, through befriending them, inner conflicts can be ended, new coping-strategies offered and inner peace found. This explanation always provokes an 'Aha Effect'. Even colleagues from other therapeutic faculties are impressed by its simplicity and the possibilities for understanding it brings to phenomena such as countertransference, our shadow and the higher aspirations in our psyche.

The Egg provides a very helpful picture of the strategies we develop to cope with life and our store of personal experiences and memories become clearer. In this realm of the Egg we work with the memory of the body, the brain and sometimes at the depth of the cellular level.

Contact with Material from Outside – Regression and Past Life Work

During therapeutic work I have observed that, when the client sees and transforms old personal patterns, a channel or connection to the Higher Self is activated and with that an openness to material that seemingly comes from former lifetimes. Without being intended, by me as the therapist or by the client, spontaneous pictures arise, which, at first sight, have nothing to do with this lifetime. These images open up a symbolic way for clients to understand their situation, enabling disidentification on a much wider scale to take place. These pictures and the distance of centuries can even enable us to look at very dark material.

I am not a Buddhist and I do not care if there are such things as personal former lifetimes or if we just 'download' symbolic and meaningful experiences from the Collective Unconscious that help us to a better understanding of our problems in this life. As long as it helps it does not matter for me. I was lucky to have David Bach MA from Monterey as my guide and therapist and later as my supervisor in the first years of encountering psychosynthesis. His non-judgemental openness to all that came up was so helpful. Bach called his work Karmic Psychology and he worked with a certain Regression Ritual that we later completed with a healing process.

During the almost 30 years of my life as a therapist I have found working this way has yielded many symbolic gifts for patients including:

- Further disidentification (by means of the large distance in time and place)
- Giving a broader context and perspective of the client's problem
- Release from repetitive compulsions
- Solving deep fears and phobias
- Releasing old core beliefs lead to a deep understanding of me being as I am
- Taking responsibility rather than falling into resignation

- Coming out of the victim status
- Employing ritual to heal at a deep soul level (soul loves rituals)

The more open the guide is towards past life work, the more the client dares to live it through, whereas a judgemental attitude stops the process. For a long time therapists, including psychosynthesis practitioners, kept their distance to this kind of work. More recently, however, we have been confronted with a real boom in 'regression and reincarnation' literature, with the market becoming flooded with books on the subject. Even famous Jungian therapists and psychiatrists such as the late Roger Woolger (1987, 2004) and Brian Weiss (1988, 1992) have written several best-sellers on the subject. It seems as if material from this realm is longing for expression, 'soul-memory' wants to be seen.

So What Keeps Us from Working this Way?

As therapists we always try to be intellectually accepted. And to me Psychosynthesis even strives harder for that acceptance. "Where is the scientific proof?" is always the question.

But how will you ever prove – with tests and questionnaires – people's experiences with inner pictures and symbols which shrink when you try to put them into words which are already secondary symbolizations. From experience – to picture – to word is the inner way. Experiences are always diminished and cut smaller by words. The biblical pronouncement "In the beginning was the word!" (John 1:1) should perhaps also be questioned: is that true or is it also only another male fiction from a churchman?

I Would Like to Invite You Even Further Out or Further Down: Into the Collective Unconscious

Since Jung proclaimed the Collective Unconscious over 70 years ago, little has been written and even less research done in this field. The roots of Collective

Unconscious lie in an archaic-mythological thinking and refer to humanity's inheritance, the store of its history which provides the psychic ground of every human being. And very like the biological body developed by evolution, formed and imprinted by its experiences, the Collective Unconscious has become a component of the whole species. While we find inside the Egg at the personal level behavioural and coping patterns that have been built as answers to shock and trauma or just to manage life, so is outside in the Collective Unconscious the memory of whole humanity with its shocks and traumata is stored.

In our training at the Circadian Institute, when we teach the Egg Diagram and we describe what is outside the dashes, I say always: You must imagine there the Collective Unconscious, the store of humanity's experience which is passed down through the ages in myth, legends and fairy tales. This realm seems to be the home of the archetypes, basic psychic pattern of humanity. Archetypes would be then 'inhabitants' of the Collective Unconscious and we could understand them as being similar to subpersonalities.

CG Jung (1984) postulates that the frequent and persevering psychic patterns which form basic pattern or archetypes also structure the psyche of the individual as well. They are numinous, having an involuntary power that the individual psyche cannot resist. Jung sees the appearance of motifs in fairy tales, myth, dreams and art as proof for the existence of archetypes. Roberto Assagioli saw archetypes as living beings, each having its own wisdom, and expressing qualities such as Beauty, Energy and Love.

Stanislav Grof (2011) said: "We are approaching a level of archetypal consciousness", meaning that we are going towards a kind of world-consciousness. Out of my 18 years of working with mythology I feel forced to change the sentence into: 'Archetypes are approaching us to change our consciousness'. I could make an analogy to my therapy sessions: during a session subpersonalities sometimes call strongly for our attention. When several clients present the same problem in therapy, it is time for me to have a session with my supervisor to clear my 'stuff' and make sense of the emerging pattern!

Something Wants to be Seen!

If we ask "What, in the outside world, wants to be seen so terribly urgently at this moment?" we are given many hints. The lies and untruthfulness we live surrounded by come more and more to the surface. 'Wikileaks', 'Vaticanleaks' and Edward Snowdon's revelations are good examples for this trend. Truth wants to be seen. Lies show up in all areas, uncovered by courageous people who are questioning politics, business and capitalism. The fictional visions of Huxley's *Brave New World*, Bradbury's *Fahrenheit 451* and Orwell's *Nineteen Eighty Four* have long been overtaken by everyday life. Are we ready to listen and to take responsibility for this? That is what the Collective seems to be asking from us at the moment.

So the logical question is how can we work in and with this realm? Archetypal Psychosynthesis seemed to me the answer.

What do We Mean by Archetypal Psychosynthesis?

We have to approach the Collective, this realm beyond or outside our personal psyche, with even greater care and a more respectful attitude than we would our subpersonalities, in order to find answers to these more planetary issues. As with the human body, the need for healing is shown by the symptoms, in this case strife, greed, war....Healing on this wider plane, then, requires the same willingness for change, openness and responsibility for our own actions as would be the case in addressing personal symptoms,

How I Came into Contact with This Realm

It started with my first visit to Ireland in 1994. In this country the 'veils' between realities seem to be very thin. Coming across mythological sites by chance I had strong experiences and 'knew' instantly what had happened in these places. Only later I learned by studying the history of the places, by reading the myths, that my 'knowing' had substance. The occurrences (sometimes battles, murder or deceit) seemed to be imprinted in the earth, in the landscape. Is there such a thing as memory of a place, akin to Rupert Sheldrake's Morphogenetic Fields? The memory of the place seemed to be talking to me. First I doubted my mind. Then I sought a quiet place to integrate the experiences and later to read all I could get about Irish Mythology.

When you reach into the realms of Mythology and Archetypes you have to go deep down and under the 'official, correct' historical record. "Dive behind and go deep down", as Mary Ellen Carne put it in her talk at the World Conference of Psychosynthesis in San Diego in 1996. It is a good advice, because the stories were passed on in oral tradition and had been deformed and then quite distorted by being written down from the 8th Century onwards by Christian monks. And we know what that means. The mythological figures were pressed into a total different value system.

A few years later I brought participants in my workshops to the same world-history soaked places. Without having been given any previous information they had the same deep experiences as I had. Now, after a long time of working with 'root-myths' in many different countries I know: touching and exploring the field 'outside', going deep into the collective experiences is enriching and life-enhancing as more levels of consciousness are discovered.

But the main question was and still is: Is there something that needs healing? How could healing be possible? And how can we be of help?

My experience was that there were always spells and curses in the myths that needed to be healed and resolved. The history of mankind is up to now HIS-story; HER-story has never been written. But we need the feminine goddess consciousness to find different models for peacemaking and reconciliation, releasing the potential that is stored in the collective unconsciousness. Healing our divine Anima, releasing feminine qualities could heal national patterns as well.

So Archetypal Psychosynthesis means going back to our imprinted world heritage, to the wisdom of our souls. It brings us back to the humbleness of medieval mystics accepting experiences that our language is too limited to put it into words. World soul wisdom asks us to no longer be ashamed of such childlike simplicity. We stand in a long tradition and could know better about our interconnectedness and oneness on this universal level:

- 2500 years ago Buddha taught the unity of all living beings
- 2000 years ago Jesus Christ told us: "We are all children of God, we are one"
- Almost 100 years ago, long before Transpersonal Psychology claimed it, Assagioli had insights about our oneness
- Over 80 years ago, Jung calling it the 'Numinous' and postulated Archetypes and Collective Unconscious as the place of our common heritage
- Over 80 years ago, Quantum Physics, as the physics of relationship, proved that the observer changes the observed object. Imagine: What that means for our work as therapists. What real influence we have: how I look at someone already changes him. And what responsibility that means as well

I recently came across a book about an exchange of letters between one of the greatest Quantum Physicists, Wolfgang Pauli and CG Jung (Meier, 2007) Pauli, like most of the great physicists came to a point in his life when he became spiritual: there is something greater behind everything, something that cannot be described. Pauli and Jung discussed the Collective Unconscious, archetypes and working on the idea of synchronicity. Pauli had many dreams about his 'Inner Magician' and alchemy, and also undertook a course of psychoanalysis. Both were greatly interested in the connections and parallels between Quantum Physics and psychology, Pauli saying: "What is still older is always the newer" (*ibid*, 2007).

Nowadays, we were so happy when Neurobiology and Neuropsychology provides proof that supports our work: demonstrating how the brain works, how we learn, how enthusiasm is fertilizing learning processes and especially how we process inner pictures into our cells and influence cell-functions with thoughts, thus demonstrating the effectiveness of Psychosynthesis interventions. We have learned about mirror neurons and other resonating phenomena: I feel what you feel. We have learned about our connectedness – our influencing each other – about the implied truth, the permeable lines of our Egg Model shows!

How Could We Work in This Area and What Could be the Benefits?

Firstly, some precautions you have to keep in mind:

1 *Mind how I look' at the client*: My eyes tell the truth: giving the client credit or looking at him with fearful eyes, through the lens of statistics, telling him with my eyes about the hopelessness of the diagnosis. It is dripping out of my pores. And it is reaching him.
2 *Mind my words*: The so-called Nocebo Effect (Latin for 'I will harm') has been the object of recent research. Opposite to the Placebo effect, where sugar pills have healing effects, it suggests that negative messages can harm or kill the person receiving them. Perhaps we should stop reading the information on the side-effects of our medicine to avoid this!
3 *Mind my thoughts:* I have responsibility not only for my looking, speaking and doing – but for my thinking as well. Although there is not as yet scientific evidence of the impact of our thoughts on others, the permeability of the Egg-Diagram we can be sure that there is an influence. Even if we do not belief in that, we should take responsibility for what we put into the 'net'

How Can Archetypal Psychosynthesis Help Us in Our Work?

To know mythology is to know the history of humanity. By 'diving in' – finding places, finding wounds, finding curses, finding treasures and releasing the wisdom and healing potential with the tools of Psychosynthesis – we could serve the well-being of our planet. Taking myths serious will sometimes unlock the truth of a place's history: Heinrich Schliemann took the writing of Homer very seriously and, as a result, discovered the objective, touchable treasures of ancient Troy. But less tangible treasures could also be found such as solving the karma of entire nations.

All over the world we can find sure signs of the unreleased history of nations and the healing needed in centuries-old grudges and successive wars fought for long forgotten reasons. Ireland is a good example, the enmity between the Singhalese and Tamil people in Sri Lanka, the isle of light, is another. In each mythology we always find treachery and a curse.

The way out is to first pacify the archetypal figures involved in a symbolic way. The work will open us more and more to the thought of unity and oneness, for our interconnectedness. Our contact to this realm has to be respectful, humble and with the innocence of a beginners mind. One of my teachers Jungian Gregg Furth warned us in our training: "They (the Archetypes) can kill you".

The gains are manifold:

- In accepting this interconnectedness we accept our power
- Loneliness changes to connectedness
- Division and separation is loss of paradise
- Fear, competition and mistrust no longer rule
- I am more than myself – I go over my borders – there is boundless plenty
- Energy is generated by remembering and releasing old patterns
- Core wounds I brought into this life are healed
- National wounds can be healed
- We have the choice what we teach: fear or love

I think time is pushing us: we have to make a decision. Do we together want to survive collectively or collectively cease to exist in the madness of envy, greed and war? With Psychosynthesis we have the means to choose. Transformation can happen through a whole variety of techniques and exercises. Our choice is to work for:

- Peace of heart
- Peace of soul
- Peace in the world

In her novel *Miriam* (1984) Marie-Luise Rinser lets Jesus say to Mary Magdalen : "Go ahead, teach the oneness of all living beings – teach love". That could be our credo.

The Hourglass Model (Brode's Enlarged Egg Diagram)

When I tried to give my experiences a visible form what emerged looked like an hourglass – the hourglass of our lifetime and beyond. I drew a three level Egg Diagram to show the different layers of therapeutic effect:

1 Inside the Egg – personal history and memories
2 Up to the Higher Self – transpersonal history and memories
3 Collective Unconsciousness – universal history and divine memory

Level of Effect
in Psychosynthesis
© Dr Kristina Brode

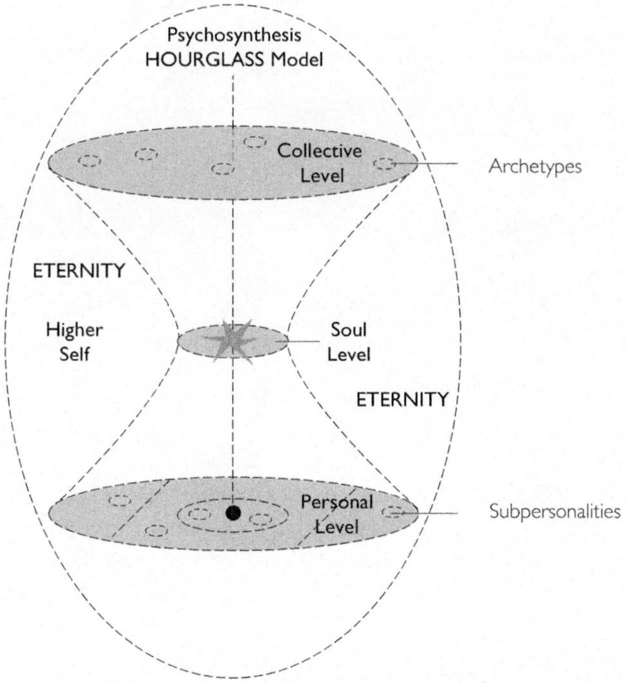

The three layers are surrounded by Eternity, as it soon became clear to me that our time is embedded in eternity – in GOD.

My curiosity does not stop here. I would like to invite you to take some risks:

- Risk thinking outside the box
- Risk seeming simple-minded
- Risk loving and see what happens

Evolution is provocation. I hope I have provoked you.

References

Assagioli, R, *CG Jung and Psychosynthesis*. Available from www.synthesiscenter.org/articles/0119.pdf

Brode, K, *Angst als Chance, Diagnose Krebs: Brücken zur Selbstheilung und einem neuen Lebensgefühl, Ein Ratgeber für Krebspatienten*, Scorpio-Verlag, 2013

Carne, ME, *Talk at the World Conference of Psychosynthesis*, San Diego, 1996

Furth, G, *Jungian Art Therapist Training Lecture*, 1983-88

Furth, G, *The Secret World of Drawings: Healing Through Art*, Sigo Press, 1988

Grof, S, *Holotopic Breathwork Seminar*, Spain, April 2011

Jung, CG, *Archetyp und Unbewusstes*, Gesamtwerk Bd 2, Walter Verlag, 1984

Meier, CA (ed.), *Atom and Archetype: The Pauli/Jung Letters from 1932-1958*, Princeton University Press, 2007

Rinser, L, *Mirjam*, Fischer Verlag, 1984

Weiss, BL, *Many Lives, Many Masters*, Simon & Schusters, 1988

Weiss, BL, *Through Time into Healing*, Fireside, 1992

Woolger, R, *Other Lives, Other Selves: A Jungian Psychotherapist Discovers Past Lives*, Doubleday, 1987

Woolger, R, *Healing Your Past Life*, Sounds True Inc., 2004

Odysseus's Blunder – The Self in the 'Mistake'

Steve Simpson

Out beyond ideas of wrong-doing and right-doing, there is a field. I'll meet you there. When the soul lies down in that grass, the world is too full to talk about. Ideas, language, even the phrase 'each other' doesn't make any sense. (Rumi, trans. Barks, 1995, p36)

Prelude

Error, mistake, wrongness, slip, bungle, cock-up, gaffe, indiscretion, etc., etc. *ad nauseam* – our language is rich in words to describe the act of blundering; rich also in habitual reactions ranging from blame and shame to cover-up and denial. The conventional attitude to blundering is, by and large, to consider it as an aberration in the 'normal' flow of events, to be corrected and avoided in future. We become transfixed by *why* we stumble, yet seldom enquire *for what*? As Rumi observes "The eye goes blind when it only wants to see *why*" (1995, p. 166). *Why*, perhaps, perpetuates the illusion that we are really in control, that if only we understood better, we could save ourselves from repeating our errors. For all the 'naming and shaming', the preoccupation with causality, still we blunder, often with catastrophic costs at the personal, collective and planetary levels. Yet despite its ubiquity the *phenomenon* of the Blunder as a feature of human life, it is seldom considered in psychological and psychospiritual literature and enquiry.

Culturally, our blunders often evoke the spirit of the Harpy, the harsh, shrieking creatures of mythology that seek to keep us 'safe' by making us fearful and cautious. In Philip Pullman's *The Amber Spyglass* (2000), the heroine, Lyra, an accomplished and imaginative liar, is confronted by a similarly malevolent Harpy and learns she can pacify her attacker only by telling the *truth*. This set me wondering about the deeper truth that gets missed when we attend to our blunders only from a place of criticism and humiliation. What, psychospiritually, do we blunder *for*? Could our mistakes, rather than presenting us with reminders of our individual and collective failings and limitations, be, instead, evidence of a higher, deeper intelligence in action? This paper sets out to explore this territory, from a psychospiritual perspective, wondering how the mistake may have a valuable function to play in personal growth and the evolution of consciousness and what it may have to teach us about the nature of Self. As our guide we will take that most complex and human of classical heroes – and epic blunderer – Homer's Odysseus (1992).

Odysseus's Blunder

I am in the hands of the unknown God,
he is breaking me down to his own oblivion
to send me forth on a new morning, a new man
(DH Lawrence, *Shadows*, 1972, p. 250)

John Ayto (1990, p. 69) defines the original meaning of the word 'blunder' as to "stumble around blindly, bumping into things" (in this we can differentiate the blunder from that other sort of transgression, the *conscious* breaking of a personal or societal moral or law – blundering, by definition, puts us into the territory of the unintended or unconscious). On the face of it Odysseus, as we come to know him through Homer's storytelling in *The Iliad* and *Odyssey*, appears to be the antithesis of a blunderer. He's a really smart guy, renowned and celebrated throughout the known world for his intelligence and cunning – and he knows it. Thinking psychologically, we could say that Odysseus is strongly identified with his 'adaptive self', the persona his psyche has adopted in order to survive and then succeed in the environment into which he was born – an age, perhaps like our own, on the cusp of profound transformation (the Age of the Hero, of brutal machismo and colonial wars, in about to give way to an era of fledgling civic and communal values).

At the outset of the events described in *The Odyssey* Odysseus is at the zenith of his career as ultimate trickster. After ten years of gruelling siege the city of Troy has finally fallen, duped into letting its defences down by Odysseus's ruse of the great wooden horse, left apparently as a peace offering by the departing Greek forces but harbouring within in it the strike force that will bring death and destruction down on the Trojans. In the aftermath of this triumph, two week's sailing will bring Odysseus safely home to his island kingdom of Ithaca and his beloved wife Penelope and son Telemachus. Yet at his moment of greatest triumph, the wily 'man of ways', so trusting of his own cleverness, commits an elementary and apparently catastrophic Blunder.

The journey homewards lies due west. Instead Odysseus, his adaptive self bloated by success, and eager to add to the loot he has already plundered from defeated Troy, takes his fleet south for what he expects to be a simple piracy raid on the seaside village of Ismarus. The familiar refrain of the addictive personality perhaps: just one more adventure, one more piece of contraband, then he heads for home and normality. It will be another ten years before Odysseus, by now utterly transformed, reaches home.

Initially the raid on Ismarus goes according to plan – another round of rape and pillage, another dose of suffering meted out to the innocent. His galleys filled with loot and slaves, Odysseus heads out for home, only to be caught up in a terrible storm. Ships, men and plunder are lost, the remainder of the fleet blown wildly off course. Already on the verge of the unknown, out of his depth psychologically, Odysseus and his comrades fetch up on the island of Polyphemus, a one-eyed Cyclops – to escape his cannibalistic attentions Odysseus outwits and kills the giant only to draw the wrath of the sea-God Poseidon, Polyphemus's uncle, who now curses the voyage with further disasters. Over the following ten years, Odysseus's' 'adaptive self' is systematically stripped away through a series of transformatory losses: he is shipwrecked more than once, blown thousands of miles off course when in sight of home, seduced and entranced by witches and nymphs, travels down into the gloom of Hades, the Underworld. And whilst on occasions he can still draw on cunning to aid survival, he is increasingly broken down and humbled by the forces of transformation unleashed on him by the gods. By the time he eventually washes ashore on Ithaca and, in the rags of a beggar, reclaims his family and kingdom, we see an Odysseus who has lived the truth of 'suffering meaning' – the 'moral imperative' that demands that ultimately we cannot avoid the call of Self – and, transcending at last his partial, limiting adaptive identification, has stepped into his full authority as father, husband, king and human being: the 'I/Self'.

Given where Odysseus is taken and the psychological transformation wrought on him, we can see that his initial mistake at Ismarus, far from being an aberration, is absolutely *necessary* in order to jolt him from his self-satisfied 'known' and into the journey of transformatory crisis and deep initiation in order for him to fulfil the potential of *who he most truly is*. This is "the Call as Blunder" which Jean Houston speaks of (1984, p. 85). Odysseus has not consciously summoned up or chosen this journey nor can he, for a very long time, hear the Call of Self encoded in the blundering that kick-started it. Indeed, for much of the story, he actively resists, clinging on to his old identity as fervently as, at one point, he hangs on to a plank of wood, all the remains of his once-proud fleet, as he is buffeted by the wild sea. He plots and laments, but ultimately knows that he must surrender to and co-operate with forces far great and wiser then himself.

Self as Blunder

From a psychosynthesis perspective we can understand Odysseus's Blunder, the doorway through which he must pass in order for transformation to happen, as the work of Self. It is almost as if Self has worked *through* the adaptive self, used it *against itself* to trick the Trickster onto a necessary path of growth and spiritual awakening.

At first glance the concept of the Blunder appears antithetical to the spirit of psychospiritual psychology, where so much of our attention is drawn to potential and transcendence. One of the great attractions of psychosynthesis as a psychology of hope is that it offers tools to transcend the mess, pain and confusion experienced at the Lower Unconscious level. Although Assagioli warns that the "spiritual is a long and arduous adventure through strange lands full of surprises, joy and beauty, difficulties and even dangers" (1993, p. 39) our personalities can easily become transfixed by what could be described as a 'Transpersonal Super-ego' which becomes frustrated and harshly critical when our personal or spiritual efforts fall short or fail to deliver us to the promised nirvana.

Psychosynthesis practitioners at all levels of experience can, periodically, find themselves weighed down, shamed and disheartened by their perceived short-comings and errors. As we peer upwards towards the Olympian heights of the possible, we can slip too readily into intolerance of our 'failings' and, by extension, our clients' lack of psychological and spiritual 'progress' (I would differentiate here between an ego-attachment to spiritual perfection/salvation and the soul's 'suffering meaning' as, through existential shame, we contemplate the gap between our Self-connected aspirations and our human limitedness). Alongside this there is often a fantasy that *if only* we could have been saved from the wounds of conception, birth and early life (i.e. the blunders and worse of parents, caregivers and environment) a sort of Eden would prevail out of which a life free of suffering would be made possible.

The Blunder reminds us of our limitations, even as we aspire for the whole, inevitably evoking the voices of judgement and humiliation that we have internalised throughout life. But what if the converse was also at play here? When, on our life's adventure, we become stuck (in a tenacious maintaining cycle or pernicious compulsion or addiction), when we cannot think or our thinking is caught in the sway of the ego, superego, adaptive self or narcissistic wound (for example, Odysseus's rigid adherence to his Trickster identity), perhaps the only way that Self can break through *is* to manufacture the Blunder. In Houston's concept of the 'Sacred Wound' (1987), a rent in the fabric of the known, however painful, is often required for what she calls the Larger Story – the sacred, collective unconscious – to enter into the everyday human realm. The Self-inspired Blunder, unwittingly committed by the personality, is one such psychospiritually necessary wound.

Furthermore, a 'wholeness' that excludes mistakes and imperfection is, by definition, *not* Whole. As Houston (*ibid*, p. 105) points out, a sacred wound evokes *pathos* – *com*passion, the opening of the heart, is called out as we suffer the consequences of our limitations in the face of our often unachieved potential: "The wounding pathos…may contain the seeds of healing and transformation… (it) becomes *sacred* when we are willing to release our old stories and to become vehicles through which the new story may emerge into time" (*ibid*, p. 105). As we know from our clinical practice to sit, heart open, with another in their shame, humiliation, self-disgust, self-attack requires as Act of Will; in our consciously chosen, Self-informed response to the Blunder – our own and the other's – the marriage of Love and Will can be birthed.

The Ethical Call

From bitter searching of the heart,
Quickened with passion and with pain
We rise to play a greater part.

This is the faith from which we start:
Men shall know commonwealth again
From bitter searching of the heart.
(Frank Scott, *Villanelle for Our Time*, 2004)

For all that we can revision the Blunder, understanding it as a mechanism by which Self breaks through into an otherwise 'stuck' consciousness, calling out a more thoughtful, compassionate , soulful response to our lapses, we must take care not to become sanguine. To do so would deny the truth that *Blunders do harm* – and that we have a moral personal responsibility in relation to our blundering, personal and collective, and its often catastrophic consequences in terms of human suffering (as witnessed in the daily reportage of persecution and injustice, poverty and famine, environmental neglect and exploitation, corporate greed and political malfeasance, the apparently perpetual addiction to warfare as a way of achieving peace).

A Self-informed response to the Blunder requires something radically different from contemporary society's habitual reaction. We seem to be gripped by a thriving 'blame culture', in which a barely conscious drive demands the 'naming and shaming' of those perceived to 'guilty' of mistakes and transgressions large and small against the collective 'good' (this could be understood as primitive, atavistic, 'magical thinking' at play, the sacrifice necessary to ward off similar future mistakes). At the intrapsychic level, this manifests as superego or a 'judge/critic' subpersonality which almost inevitably has its polarity in a 'victim' part. Although this could be seen as a limited if flawed attempt at 'moral being', its effect is almost always regressive. When blame and shame are directed outwardly the heart and mind close and the opportunity for deeper understanding lost. When these energies are inwardly directed the will can become frozen, hooked into cycles of self-recrimination, re-enforcing the identity with the wounds of history and re-enacting the critical self-deflating messages of history. Odysseus presents what could be seen as the opposite side of the 'narcissistic split' to this as he seems oblivious, at least initially, to the terrible cost both to himself and others of his actions – for all his 'cleverness' he lacks the capacity for self-reflection.

Miles Davis, the great jazz trumpeter, tells us "Do not fear mistakes – there are none" (quoted in Cameron, 1994, p. 194). My sense of what he means by this is that the apparent Blunder, if responded to with openness, can provide the unexpected note from which a glorious new improvisation can develop. This requires *mastery*: not only technical skill (Miles, like all great improvisers, had to master his scales before his music could take flight) but other attributes – attentiveness, flexibility and the humility to surrender to, be carried by and act as the servant of a force greater than oneself. Applied more broadly and drawing on a psychospiritual sensibility, we could understand the mistake as requiring an *ethical response* from us. I would argue that this means not falling back into a guarded, cautious position, where we are constantly 'red alert' and will freezes as a consequence (or worse, a rigid form of self-righteousness and moralism takes hold). Nor is it as simple as being willing to learn from our mistakes, especially if in doing so we merely reinstate the previous status quo which, temporarily at least, the Blunder has jolted out of its well-worn groove – what needs to be learnt is a new methodology of response ('response-ability' more than responsibility?) Key to this is *reflection* – the willingness to 'press the pause button', take a step back and wonder at what is being presented or seeking to emerge (this, it seems to me, lies at the heart of supervision of our clinical practice, especially when holding a psychospiritual context). A challenging but essential aspect of this reflective process is what Scott calls "bitter searching of the heart" (*ibid*, 2004) and the 12 Step Programme's 'deep moral inventory', a conscious and honest engagement with what has happened and our part it in it. In this, there must be space for remorse (opening the heart to the impact, the cost, to self and other); contrition (heartfelt sorrow, 'pathos' once again) and reparation (a commitment to Acts of Will that can be both reparative and transformatory). Each of these actions – moral imperatives – is properly the territory of the awakened 'I'. Beyond this, opening to Self, we need to stay curious to the Call whispering through the symptom of the Blunder.

The Blunder in the Therapy Room

The puzzle in therapy is not how did I get this way, but what does my angel want with me? (Hillman, 1992, p. 70)

I was tempted to call this section 'the therapist as blunderer'. The shadows of failure – missing our clients, evoking their disappointment or rage, re-wounding, acting out our frustration/ anger/desire, not-knowing (our 'expertise' exposed as empty-handed wizardry), professional censure, a malpractice suit – all haunt the recesses of the therapy room. Yet hour-on-hour, one way or another, we blunder along, often in a state of 'not knowing'. Though we do our best, endeavouring to disidentify, remain grounded in I/Self, 'turning up, not retaliating and not falling asleep' the Blunder inevitably barges its way in. And not just the practitioners' Blunder: it is often a blunder that propels the client into therapy – the mistake that has brought their psychological walls crashing down; the error repeated with devastating effect in the form of addiction, compulsive behaviour or adherence to a fruitless maintaining cycle; the impact of what could be termed 'life's blunder' (bereavement, abuse, mortal illness, loss of career, failure of relationship). There is also the Blunder where the client comes for the 'wrong' thing, for instance as when, through the therapeutic process, the apparently simple initial presenting issue is stripped away to reveal far deeper wound, crisis or call.

In the spirit of Rumi's poem *Guest House* (Kornfield, 2000, p. XI), in which he imagines the arrival of the "unexpected visitor" who will "violently sweep your house empty of its furniture…clearing you out for some new delight", can we honour the Blunder when it manifests in the consulting, welcome it "as a guide from beyond"? As therapists can we embody 'mastery' not as a form of error-resisting control, but in the manner of Miles Davis, with awareness, respect, open-heartedness, flexibility, curiosity and imagination? Can we hold a context in which we regard the Blunder as "necessary, a way soul enters the world, a way the soul gains truths that could not be encountered through reason alone" as Hillman (1975, p. 160) urges, (he goes on to tell us that "(p)sychological awareness rises from errors, coincidences, indefiniteness, from the chaos deeper than intelligent control" (*ibid*, p. 160).

The following brief vignettes demonstrate the transformative value and power of welcoming and being with (rather than seeking to eradicate) the Blunder in the therapy room.

• • •

Diane and Martin – 'Mastery' in the Face of the Blunder

Diane, a highly committed and responsible trainee therapist taking her first steps as a clinician, books in an appointment to see her new client Martin at 5pm on the Wednesday following their initial consultation. At 5.15 on the appointed day, Diane, immersed in writing a paper for her course, suddenly and shockingly remembers that at that very moment she should be meeting her client. Her initial horror gives way to panic and guilt. What should she do? She contemplates lying to Martin, inventing a story that will excuse her and rescue him from feeling 'forgotten'. As she sits with her dilemma, breathes and disidentifies, Diane sees she must tell him the truth, apologise and take responsibility for her Blunder. She calls Martin, owns up to forgetting, offers no excuses and rebooks the appointment for the following week. Even in the grip of her shame, Diane is able to notice that Martin seems more relieved than – as she had feared – angry with her: relieved that nothing bad had happened to her and also that the missed session was not down to an error of his making. Nonetheless, Diane approaches the next meeting with some trepidation. However, unpacking what has happened Martin expresses his gratitude for Diane's willingness to be honest with him about her mistake and not attempt to fob him off or pass the blame onto him. In this, Diane's response provided a huge contradiction to the experience of Martin's 'Child of History' and created the ground for a deeper trust and effective 'therapeutic alliance' to form. As the work unfolded, Martin was able to explore how he went 'missing' to/forgot himself in relationship; and, through supervision, Diane was able to understand her Blunder in terms of counter transference.

Jerry and Beryl – 'Right' Therapy for the 'Wrong' Reasons

Jerry's therapy with Beryl illustrates the Blunder at work at a number of levels. Jerry contacts Beryl wanting to work on his 'creative block' as a painter. Beryl, who has unrealised creative ambitions of her own, is excited to have the opportunity to facilitate what she sees the emergence of Jerry's creativity, initially missing the extent that he is wounded and his will caught. As their work together progresses other issues emerge: Jerry is entirely dependent on the income of his partner, who is a successful corporate lawyer, to support his art; during the hours of the day when he could be researching and working on his novel, is often stoned or drunk; and embarks on a sexual liaison with a neighbour. The focus of the sessions gradually shifts to tracking Jerry's maintaining cycles, though he remains stuck, his 'I' determinedly as yet unawakened. Then life blunders in: Alex, Jerry's highflying partner suffers a health crisis and is diagnosed with a debilitating chronic illness that requires she resigns from her job. In the crisis Beryl is finally able to engage with Jerry's sense of purpose and will. They explore what is called for from Jerry in the face of his partner's illness and the threat to their financial secu-

rity. Jerry awakens to the 'I/Self', though not in the grand romantic manner he (and his therapist) had imagined when their context was his creative block. He ends his affair, curtails his drinking and deletes his dope dealer's number from his phone – then sets about finding a job. The work he gets as a teaching assistant in an infant school, far humbler than his grand yet unembodied artistic ambitions, is of genuine service and in it Jerry begins to find himself genuinely fulfilled and purposeful for the first time in his life.

Jude and William – Discovering the Voice of this Calling Through the Blunder

Jude, a woman in her mid-forties, has come adrift from her life. Her marriage of many years has broken down, partly, as she recognises, due to her identification with a rampant, angry 'Judge' subpersonality. Now she is embroiled in a bitter divorce and custody battle and the business she and her husband had built together has collapsed. In desperation she takes the recommendation of a close friend and books in to see William, an experienced psychosynthesis therapist. Jude has never heard of psychosynthesis and has only a passing interest in questions of meaning, soul and spirit. What she wants is someone to listen to her and help her untangle the mess of her life. One day in William's waiting room Jude picks up and reads a flier advertising a 'Fundamentals of Psychosynthesis' intensive. A bell rings for her: although she cannot fully articulate it, she is aware of a beauty that draws her, especially in the idea that she might be more than her wounded behaviour, that there could be potential and meaning in her present suffering. Attending the Fundamentals weekend sets Jude on an utterly expected course, not only of deep personal transformation but of responding to a vocational call to service, to train and practice as a psychospiritual psychotherapist. Now hugely experienced in second career, Jude still meets with William from time to time and they both look back with a sense of wonder at how her Blunder led to her finding her true calling in life.

The Blunder: Stumbling – Or Pushed – Into Grace?

We, like Odysseus, sail off to Ismarus again and again, persisting in automatic behaviour. The inevitable results help us accumulate a store of disasters that will eventually create the stimulus for change. (Houston, 1984, p. 84)

In a sense we are all Odysseus, attached to the known, putting our best foot forward but often groping blindly in the dark. We trip, fall, pick ourselves up, brush ourselves of...and, hopefully, rather than having to start all over again, our consciousness shifts and more of the erstwhile slumbering 'I/Self' becomes available to us.

If, as Emmylou Harris sings we "...stumble into grace" (2003), it seems as if Self, commandeering the stuck maintaining cycle or momentary lapse into blindness to its own purposes, does the tripping. In much the same way that Odysseus's journey of initiation and transformation is actively influenced by spirit, as represented by the Olympian gods, so it appears as if the wounded, fragmented, slumbering psyche has to be, on occasion, pushed, pulled, nudged and sometimes tricked so that it can be a more awake vehicle for Self to be manifested in life.

We come full circle, back to Odysseus, supremely confident in his concrete mind, his known world, about to be tripped into the Blunder by which he will be, through a series of wonderful and terrible encounters, adventures and losses, be stripped down in order to awaken and live from his deepest 'I/Self' nature.

References

Assagioli, R, *Psychosynthesis: A Manual of Principles and Techniques*, Aquarian/Thorson, 1993

Ayto, J, *Bloomsbury Dictionary of Word Origins*, Bloomsbury, 1990

Cameron, J, *The Artist's Way*, Souvenir Press, 1994

Hillman, J, *Revisioning Psychology*, Harper Perennial, 1975

Hillman, J and Ventura, M, *We've Had a Hundred Years of Psychotherapy and the World's Getting Worse*, Harper, 1992

Harris, E, *O Evangeline, On Stumble into Grace*, Nonesuch Records, 2003 (music CD)

Houston, J, *The Search for the Beloved*, Crucible, 1987

Houston, J, *The Hero and the Goddess*, Aquarian/Thorsons, 1992

Kornfield, J, *After the Ecstasy, the Laundry*, Rider, 2000

Lawrence DH, *Selected Poetry*, Penguin, 1972

Rumi, 'Someone Digging in the Ground' in *The Soul is Here for its Own Good*, Bly R, (ed.), The Ecco Press, 1995

Rumi, *The Essential Rumi*, Coleman Barks (trans.) with John Moyne, AJ Arberry and Reynold Nicholson, HarperOne, 2004, 1995

Scott, F, 'Villanelle for Our Time' on *Dear Heather*, Cohen, L, Columbia, 2004 (music CD)

Wider Perspectives

Psychosynthesis and Our Sacred Earth

Molly Young Brown

Our separation from the natural world may have given us the fruits of technology and science, but it has left us bereft of any instinctual connection to the spiritual dimension of life – the connection between our soul and the soul of the world, the knowing that we are all part of one living, spiritual being. (Llewellyn Vaughan-Lee)

How can the spiritual psychology of psychosynthesis help meet the challenges of the 21st century? The chaotic effects of climate change are impacting life around the Earth, brought on by human greed and self-centeredness. Radical change is upon us, along with the suffering such change can bring. We will likely have to endure years and years of intermingled catastrophes, as our oil-dependent profit-centred economies unravel and collapse, clean water becomes increasingly scarce, natural disasters and epidemics sweep through the lands, untold numbers of species become extinct, desperate military interventions are attempted, and democracy struggles to survive. Add to this the likelihood of more nuclear disasters contaminating the entire planet with radioactivity, like the one still unfolding in Japan.

David Korten (2006) calls this collapse of our unsustainable economic, political, and energy systems, "the Great Unraveling". Things have gone too far for us to completely stop the process; we can only hope to slow it down and mitigate the effects. Who knows how long it will take our planet to rebalance and heal, even if we humans manage to rapidly transform our systems? Meanwhile, we see people reacting with denial and distraction, fear and anger, grasping and greed, lies and violence – thereby amplifying the downward spiral.

A psychospiritual psychology that fails to address these challenges serves more as an escape than a true spiritual path, because the underlying causes of these crises are both psychological and spiritual. They arise from our beliefs about who we are as humans and our right relationship with Earth and its myriad life forms. We have been thinking of ourselves as separate and competitive with one another and with other living beings. Some religious teachings even speak of spiritual salvation or enlightenment as something individuals can achieve on their own, separate from the rest of life around them.

Of course, everything we require for life comes from the living Earth: air, water, food, clothing, and shelter. Conditioned by the modern industrial world, we tend to forget this; we act as if humans can simply produce all we want and need out of our genius, while using Earth as supply house and sewer. This world view has resulted in enormous suffering and damage to our life support systems; it has brought us to the brink of extinction.

"The world is not a problem to be solved; it is a living being to which we belong. The world is part of our own self and we are a part of its suffering wholeness. Until we go to the root of our image of separateness, there can be no healing. And the deepest part of our separateness from creation lies in our forgetfulness of its sacred nature, which is also our own sacred nature." (Vaughan-Lee, 2013, p. 1)

There's another story that can redeem us: a story of our deep inter-connectedness and interdependence within the web of life. Psychosynthesis supports this story. In psychosynthesis, we learn to acknowledge and accept all the parts within our psyches, and work with them towards harmony and peace. We learn to disidentify from social conditioning and the effects of trauma and abuse. We can do the same in our relationships with one another and with all living systems of Earth. We can disidentify from the conditioning of our materialistic, profit-driven political economy, and consciously identify with our sacred Earth and its myriad life forms.

Roberto Assagioli spoke to this in *The Act of Will*: "Altruistic love is not limited to the members of the human family. It can also embrace all living things in the animal and vegetable kingdoms of nature. This inclusiveness is expressed in the Buddhist love for all living creatures, and by Saint Francis in his 'Song of the Creatures'.

One might say that an increasingly conscious sense of this universal brotherhood is behind the growing trend toward the cultivation of harmonious relations with the environment. This is the higher and broader aspect of ecology" (2010, p. 84). The Buddhists call this altruistic love *bodhichitta* – the fervent desire for the welfare of all beings.

The Great Turning

When we look clearly and courageously at our world today, we observe another phenomenon accompanying the Great Unraveling; we see what some call the Great Turning occurring right now all around the world, a Great Turning from the 'Industrial Growth Society' – based on profit, greed, and competition – to a 'Life Sustaining Society' – based on gratitude, love and cooperation, honouring Life itself above all else.

In our individual lives, it often takes a crisis to catalyse change. Many of us know people whose lives have been transformed by a life-threatening illness. So it is with groups of people, nations, and even humanity as a whole. At this pivotal time in human history, we walk into the unknown together, as into an initiation, a collective encounter with the human soul. We in the industrialized world have reached the end of our collective adolescence; it is time now to grow up, to move fully into true adulthood, with a broader, more encompassing sense of responsibility to the Earth, all its peoples, and all its life forms: "The global ecological crisis is also the defining spiritual crisis of the human species. We are being challenged as a species, to 'grow up or get out of the way'" (Stanley and Loy, 2013, p. 45).

Global environmental and economic crises can summon a rite of passage for humanity. We can do more than endure the dark times ahead; we can actively embrace them and use them for transformation. That's what the Great Turning is all about.

Please take a moment to think of one thing you love about life on Earth at this time. Just pick the first thing that comes to mind and let yourself feel how grateful you are for this in your life. Allow this experience of gratitude to expand your heart.

Now ask yourself 'What troubles me about the world at this time?' Let your mind survey all the destruction and violence in the world today and see what troubles you the most. Let yourself feel whatever emotions come up as you think of these things – anger, fear, numbness, and especially grief. These feelings are not neurotic; they are evidence of our healthy awareness of what is happening to our world.

We feel this anguish because we love this sacred Earth; we love Life. We love because we are all deeply interconnected within the web of life. Love and anguish are two sides of the same coin, and they are the keys to the Great Turning. We must honour and embrace our love for the sacred Earth, *and* the pain we feel at injury to its living web.

Three Dimensions of the Great Turning

Eco-philosopher Joanna Macy and I describe three mutually reinforcing dimensions of the Great Turning in our book, *Coming Back to Life* (Macy and Brown, 1998).

Perhaps the most visible dimension of the Great Turning consists of the countless actions to slow down the destruction being wrought by the Industrial Growth Society. These take political, legislative, and legal forms, and include aid to those harmed and dispossessed, as well as direct actions such as blockades, boycotts, and civil disobedience. We call them 'holding actions' because they attempt to 'hold the line' to buy time for more basic changes to take place.

The second dimension includes both the analysis of the structural and institutional causes of the problems, and the creation of alternatives. We examine, for example, the tacit agreements that create obscene wealth for a few, while progressively impoverishing the rest of humanity. We explore the interlocking causes of our entanglement in a greedy economy that destroys life-supporting ecosystems across the planet.

We are also creating systemic alternatives. In countless localities, like green shoots pushing up through the rubble, new social and economic arrangements are sprouting: community gardens, farmers' markets, bike lanes and trails, local currencies, time banks. They may be hard to see at first, because they are seldom featured in the media. Not waiting for our national or local politicos to catch up with us, we are banding together, taking action in our own communities.

The third dimension is more inward work that we can do alone and together. It includes psychological and spiritual study, processes, and practices that can bring about a shift in our world-view and values, and connect us with a source of strength, love, and courage for the challenges before us. In this third dimension, we work to change our essential world view, from 'anthropocentrism' to 'eco-centrism', from seeing humans as the centre of the world, to seeing ourselves as interconnected participants in the web of life, no more or less important than any other parts. (Yes, we may have a special role to play, but so do the decomposing bacteria that turn waste into nutrients. Think of where we would be without them!)

Many people today are engaged in at least one, if not all, of these three dimensions. All three are necessary for the creation of a sustainable civilization, and each supports and feeds the other two. For example, people who are engaged in defending a particular watershed against destructive development may have to study the history of corporations to understand why they have so much power (second dimension). They may need to deepen their sense of interconnection within the web of life, and strengthen their commitment to non-violence (third dimension).

Since before the turn of the century, and for a decade or two before that, we have seen this Great Turning happening within and around us, and it seems to be intensifying every year. We have seen a worldwide awakening of concern for the planetary environment. Many young people especially have taken up the cause of defending the environment from destruction. We have seen people rising up to claim their human rights and demand more democratic governments. We have seen the Occupy movement and Idle No More take to the streets, calling attention to the criminal behavior of many corporations and the growing economic injustice that results.

Paul Hawkin has written a book called *Blessed Unrest* about the more than 2 million grass-roots organisations and projects underway today all over the world – dedicated to restoring the environment and fostering social justice. His subtitle is: *How the Largest Movement in the World Came into Being and Why No One Saw It Coming*. He provides us with proof positive that the Great Turning is real. It is happening right now, and each of us can play a part.

However, the Great Unravelling is taking place at the same time, and we face the real possibility that our current civilization – and even the human species – will not survive. Change nearly always requires a certain amount of unravelling. I am a knitter, and often have to unravel several rows of knitting to correct an error. However, if I can't pick up the stitches after unravelling, or if I unravel too far, I may have to start over. If too much harm is done before we radically change our ways, we could be reduced to a few isolated groups of people scratching out a living from a devastated environment. The outcome of the Great Turning remains uncertain, but that doesn't mean we should give up.

Uncertainty is always part of life, especially in important transitions like birth, child rearing, marriage, or a new job. Uncertainty can bring us more fully into the present moment, awake and alert. Uncertainty can evoke our will, our vision for the world we want, and endow the present moment with meaning and purpose – all familiar concepts in psychosynthesis.

Each of us is already contributing to this Great Turning in large and small ways, perhaps some we don't even recognise. Yet we may be held back by fear, a sense of inadequacy, or confusion about how to proceed. We may feel overwhelmed by the challenges of our personal lives, with no time or energy available for action in the larger community. And the fact is we do need time for inner work on ourselves, as well as outer work in the community.

Inner psychological and spiritual work will help us make a fundamental shift to a new relationship to our planetary life support system and with the whole human family. It will help us develop Assagioli's 'broader altruistic love', the Buddhists' 'bodhichitta'. It is the work of the third dimension of the Great Turning. And I believe this is where psychosynthesis can make its greatest contribution.

The Role of Psychosynthesis

I see psychosynthesis serving the Great Turning in four powerful ways:

1. Psychosynthesis can help individuals heal the wounds from their past, wounds that create grasping, fear and confusion – what the Buddhists call the three causes of suffering. Psychosynthesis applied to counselling, psychotherapy, family therapy, addictions, and personal growth does this effectively.

2. Psychosynthesis can support us, and help us support others, through the Great Unravelling. No matter how successful we are in turning things around, many of our crises, such as climate change, cannot be stopped in their tracks. We may be able to mitigate some of the worst effects, but there *will be* very hard times ahead. We in the psychosynthesis community may be called upon to act as chaplains, to guide others through various challenges and traumas, and to teach the skills we know: centering, disidentification, self-observation, developing the will, and more.

3. Psychosynthesis can help strengthen activists who are working on the front lines, in the first and second dimensions of the Great Turning, strengthening their courage, compassion and connection to Self.

4 Psychosynthesis can contribute to the shift in consciousness we all need, away from self-centeredness and egotism, to experiencing and acting from our essential oneness in the web of life. I believe the tools of disidentification and Self-identification can help with that shift, as we expand our sense of who we are – from little monads, little embattled egos, to interconnected participants in the grand adventure of Life.

Joanna Macy (1998) calls this the "holonic shift". It's as if we are starting to think, feel and act as one larger organism, using our collective wisdom, not simply adding up yours and mine. We still act as individuals, but we sense the promptings of a larger Intelligence guiding us. Our actions arise from what deep ecologist John Seed (1988, p. 36) once described as the rain forest defending itself through us. We expand our identification from separate egos, groups, or even nations, and begin to identify as part of Ecological Self. I believe this is another name for Higher Self or Transpersonal Self. And we celebrate the diverse roles that everyone plays, including our own.

As we continue our study and practice of psychospiritual psychology, let's imagine that everything we learn can contribute to the Great Turning. How can this practice or concept or approach help us to heal old wounds that may be holding us enslaved to addictions, fear or powerlessness? How can it help to strengthen and centre us, preparing us for the challenges ahead? How can it help to expand our identification beyond our personal, social, and economic boundaries to the most inclusive, compassionate sense of Self?

We face huge and complex challenges in the coming decades, greater than any other challenges humanity as a whole has ever faced. Here we have no experts, because no one alive today has ever dealt with this enormity of change. We truly walk together into the unknown. So we must call upon our deepest spiritual resources, including the wisdom of wild nature, to guide us, moment to moment, on the journey ahead.

We have enormous capacities and resources within and around us, if we can throw off limiting beliefs and conditioning and release the power, creativity, and beauty that lie within us. We are so much stronger, so much more capable, so much wiser than we have believed up until now.

Moreover, we can draw upon the vast intelligence of Life, an intelligence that has brought us this far. Life has transformed itself through the eons of Earth's evolution, overcoming life-threatening challenges many times. We can rely on Life's vast store of wisdom and love to support us with every breath.

Help and guidance are available to us for the asking. When we don't know what to do, we can align with Self, ask for guidance and then act on it. Self is an inexhaustible Source that acts through us when we open ourselves to its energies.

May psychosynthesis contribute to the transformation of humanity and to the birth of a Life-sustaining society based on love, cooperation, and planetary health.

References

Assagioli, R, *The Act of Will*, Synthesis Center Press, 2010

Hawkins, P, *Blessed Unrest*, Viking, 2007

Korten, D, *The Great Turning: From Empire to Earth Community*, Berrett-Koehler, 2006

Macy, J, Brown, MY, *Coming Back to Life: Practices to Reconnect Our Lives, Our World*, New Society Publishers, 1998 (New edition Fall 2014)

Seed, J, Macy, J, Fleming, P and Naess, A, *Thinking Like a Mountain: Towards a Council of All Beings*, New Society Publishers, 1988

Stanley, J and Loy, D, 'At the edge of the roof: the evolutionary crisis of the human spirit', in *Spiritula Ecology: The Cry of the Earth*, The Golden Sufi Center, 2013

Vaughan-Lee, L, (ed.), *Spiritual Ecology: The Cry of the Earth*, The Golden Sufi Center, 2013

Dimensions of Difference

Keith Silvester

This is a discussion about the nature of conflict. We live in a world where differences abound. Much of the time, with enough life maturity, we come to terms with 'the otherness of the other' without coming to blows. Yet, if we take even a cursory look at our world – everything from the big global picture to our proximal, closest relationships, we see difficulty, often insurmountable. For those of us working as therapists, consultants, coaches – whether with individuals, couples, groups or organisations – we are made to engage with the nature of difference and how it escalates into conflicts of various kinds. And the conflicts do not arise simply because of people's immaturity, inaccurate perceptions or even lack of good will. Some of these conflicts, it could be argued, are inherent to the human condition. Yet others are possibly avoidable. Others are just intractable. A few years back I was struck by a particular cartoon in a magazine. It consisted of a mother looking over the shoulders of two young children very absorbed in a paper and pen exercise, while talking to another mother nearby. The caption went something like "I've set them the task of solving the Middle East problem. That will be keep them occupied for the summer holidays".

What follows is a particular framework for looking at differences, because not all differences are the same, paradoxically. The discussion will involve a psychosynthesis perspective. In so doing it will also go some way to explain why there happen to be differences within the psychosynthesis world. Close to home, in our own backyard, we have had to come to terms with splits, disagreements and fundamental antipathies – despite being intelligent, well-meaning people. How could this be? (Psychosynthesis, by the way, is certainly not unique within the therapy world for such features.)

A case in point: for many years I have belonged to a group of psychotherapists and counsellors that was set up to discuss matters of political and societal importance in the world. In the early years we would choose topics, present papers and hold robust discussions. However, in recent years certain differences have manifested within the group, and bit by bit the group has become absorbed in 'process' to try to resolve these issues. Although various people have protested that we were not set up to be a therapy group it has been become clear that our group conflicts represent a fascinating microcosm of what goes on in the outside world. If a group of educated, aware therapists cannot find a language and a method of resolving differences, how would the rest of the planet be expected to do it?

This is not a treatise on the specific practicalities of *working* with conflict. There are many methods and approaches for working with processes with people, for example, Rosenberg's Nonviolent Communication. What I am attempting to do here is to clarify three generic types of potential conflict, each arising from a 'different type of difference'. In understanding these three categories – which may or may not be exclusive and may overlap – it will point the way to strategic approaches that are helpful. I have called these categories 'dimensions', because each one has scale and size with its own implications.

Dimension I: The Great Chessboard of Life

This is the type of difference with which we are perhaps most readily familiar with. It is not hard to appreciate, at least conceptually, that each person is born into different world circumstances, has different physical makeup, genetic disposition, nutritional and health conditions. Families, communities and cultures are all different and offer specific advantages and liabilities. And of course the events we have been exposed to affect our history and the various trauma we have had to endure and overcome. So, if you are born black, disabled, working class, gay, poor – these are the features that shape your biography. Hans-Georg Gadamer in *Truth and Method* speaks of 'historically effected consciousness' where people are 'embedded' in the history and culture in which whey were shaped. Edward Said, in his 1978 book *Orientalism* put forward a view of how colonialism created a sort of 'otherness' in the mind of Europeans.

The metaphor I like to use is the chessboard. Imagine you are piece on such a board. Your function, paths of movement and rules will be different from most other pieces. From your position on one of the sixty-four squares the configuration of the board and the other pieces will be unique. Nobody else will see the positions and angles in the same way you do. Furthermore, when you or others move, the configurations and possibilities will all change. Learning to recognise and accept that the view of the chessboard and the inherent possibilities of movement will inevitably be specific and unique to each person may seem obvious in concept, but very often hard to appreciate in practice when we 'run up' against another. This is not just a problem of narcissism, but of perception and experience. The NLP idea of taking up first, second and third perceptual positions (respectively: my view, the view in someone else's shoes, and the view of the players as a whole) is helpful here. Easy perhaps, but think of just how hard it is in practice to do the simple thing of seeing the world as another sees it. As one writer put it, "don't judge a person until you have walked in his shoes for at least a mile".

Into the mix go all the prejudices and forces of habit which predispose us to react to difference without self-reflection or discrimination (in the positive sense). Much of the time, we are placed in such a position where the urgencies of life needs are simply different: for example, when we consider the arguments for and against the movement of refugees from war-torn zones, for economic migrants. People have the will to survive by whatever means they can and this can come up against the needs of others to protect what they have and not allow in 'the other'. There is the story of the two cooks fighting over a single orange. When someone came in and asked what they each wanted, one said it was the peel and the other said it was the fruit itself. In this case, the difference was resolved by identifying and respecting the need. So, some of these differences are circumstantial – and in this one might include the biological, psychological and emotional circumstances of one's origins; and others are more perceptual – how the world looks and feels from one's position.

Dimension 2: Following the Personal Star

Let us suppose that the differences discussed in Dimension 1 could be recognised, addressed and resolved. Would that mean there would now be no need for conflict? This cannot be true. We see intelligent and aware people in all walks of life disagreeing over philosophical positions, choices of direction, matters of taste, and so on. Why do I have to say "well I need to do my thing, you need to do yours"? In the psychotherapy world for example, why do organisations split from each other? Psychosynthesis is a case in point, so let's take the situation in a city like London where there are three training organisations. Although each would subscribe to some fundamental tenets of psychosynthesis (the transpersonal, the development if 'I' awareness, love and will, and so on), the style of training, the emphasis on some types of experience over others, and the body of ideas promulgated have developed very differently over time. We notice this most obviously when prospective students visit all three organisations and make choices about which training they are going to enrol on. A similar process is involved when psychotherapy students choose between one modality rather than another. This of course might simply be described as the process of individuation: people develop in different ways and follow different paths – not a strange idea to many therapeutic traditions. Or this could be framed in terms of the particular personality styles if the founders of schools and traditions. But it begs the following question: why do people individuate in the way they do? Is it all just reducible to the first dimension of that chessboard of difference described earlier?

A straightforward answer is that people have different innate talents and manifest different qualities of self. Why does Billy Elliot want to be a dancer and not a boxer, when all the circumstances of his upbringing in the more traditional North-East would lean towards the latter? He needed to follow his star, and not the star of others. We cannot fully explain why we follow our own 'star', let alone why our individual star is not the same as someone else's. But we know when we find it, and a vital part of the therapeutic process – at least for psychosynthesis, Jungians and other self-psychologies – is for the therapist to be able to acknowledge and 'meet' the other in their star in a validating way. Alas, not all therapists do this, largely because they are concerned only with ego psychology and healthy 'functioning' person in the world.

So, our own personal 'star', or what some would call our 'path', is something that we each discover in our unique way, either helped or hindered by Dimension I circumstances, or sometimes in spite of these. If we are lucky we meet people along the way who encourage us to follow our star. If we are not lucky, the will to do this has to come entirely from within. History is littered with examples of people who rejected mainstream traditions or the prevailing zeitgeist to furrow their own path. The artist Patrick Heron and the architectural commentator Ian Nairn would be possible examples. Of course, in hindsight, it is easy to congratulate such people for being true individuals. At the time though, it is often not possible to know whether this is just young, narcissistic arrogance or a response to something deeper and more profound in the calling of the self. In fiction we might be drawn to the story of *Yentl* by Isaac Bashevis Singer (which was made into the 1980s film starring Barbra Streisand) about a young Jewish woman drawn to train in rabbinics in a male-only world. These ideas are of course not new. James Hillman's 'acorn theory' and the idea of following one's personal 'daimon' are well known. Philip Pullman, in his famous His Dark Materials trilogy, even made the personal daimon into a physical creature who accompanied people.

A second take on following one's star might be a systemic one. Although we might experience our uniqueness and specific life path, we are all inextricably connected, often in ways that are unconscious. This means that each of us might be reflecting something of the whole. Although we might experience this is as 'difference' in a very separative way, there is a sort of connectivity-in-opposition. The ability to stand in the 'other' place can at times be lonely but experienced as necessary – both by the person and the society in which that person lives. For example, whatever one might have thought of leaders such as Churchill or Thatcher, they stood their ground, often in the face of opposition, and in retrospect might be seen as functional to their systems of the times in which they lived.

There is often a confusion, found even in the psychosynthesis world sometimes, between propensities and qualities. All human beings have the same propensities – we have various species-specific characteristics such as the ability to love, feel, split off painful experiences, attack, etc. However, as for qualities, well we do not always manage to develop or make the most of these. And not all people manifest the same ones.

Dimension 3: Consciousness and Maturity

This is perhaps the most difficult area to describe, and even harder to validate in any objective way. It is a dimension that is about the development of the whole human, the psychological journey, and the expansion of awareness and what we might call our Buddha nature.

There have been many attempts mapping this dimension: Ken Wilber's (2006) Integral model is one, Chris Cowan's and Don Beck's Spiral Dynamics (1996)model is another, and Robert Kegan's (1982) developmental psychology framework is a third. Although such models are used to describe individual development, they may be more frequently used to describe whole societies or even whole epochs in human culture. Models such as these have certain features in common, such as the ability to engage with and integrate complex patterns of thought, reflection and relationship.

But there are many inherent problems in any attempt to map such models of consciousness. The first is very obvious: any human being who develops a model is, by definition, not a wholly objective observer, because she or he is still part of the system being mapped. The second problem is very much a cultural one: the three models mentioned above, for example, are all western-focused and are culturally biased. In fact, it may be argued that any attempt to create a model that includes everything is risky, open to be criticised, revised, or debunked by future generations. This is inevitably the history of western thought, whether we are talking about culture, science or human growth. Other cultures may well have very different frameworks for understanding human nature and development.

There is a third problem which has a number of features making the whole enterprise of assessing human growth very complicated indeed. It is that people cannot agree on the validity of what we are looking at. For one thing, if we accept Wilber's proposition (2006) that there are different 'lines of development', each at a different stage of maturity, then we see the curious phenomenon that people are a 'mixed bag' – well developed in some respects, but not in others. In psychosynthesis terms, we have a variety of subpersonalities which have varying degrees of maturity and depth. From a postmodern, phenomenological perspective, these subpersonalities are highly mutable, and are revealed in a situationally, context-dependent way. And even if there was a certain consistency or predictability about their manifestation there is the problem of the shadow. For each of our gifts, we bring up shadow which has to be integrated into the whole personality.

A second aspect to this problem is that even if we accepted that there is a route towards self-realisation, this does not always manifest in the same way across individuals and cultures. This is perhaps most famously represented in the debate between Ferrer and Wilber, where Ferrer disputes the idea that we are akin to many rivers leading to the same ocean. Instead he posited the idea that we one ocean with many shores. In other words, not only are there many paths to enlightenment, but enlightenment looks rather different to each person when you get there! Why do I meet the symbol of a rabbi, whereas you might meet the Virgin Mary?

This aside, I do believe it is possible to suggest that there is an average 'centre of gravity' of personal development, where we move from more narcissistic and adaptive states through to being increasingly capable of being more relational and self-directed, through to being less identified with form. Another way of saying this is the typology of gross to subtle to causal to non-being. Quite how we measure this in ordinary life on an average day, with its highs, lows and frustrations is another matter!

So, the central problem with Dimension 3 is: what do we do when faced with other people whose emotional, mental and 'moral' capabilities are different from ours? What happens when a fairly 'evolved' soul encounters the 'monstrousness' of the other? Is it a recipe for conflict or for compassionate understanding? What do we do when we land up in concentration camps?

Difference, Conflict and Synthesis

When we find ourselves in conflict or simply experiencing differences – whether just between individuals or part of a couple, group or nation even – we are not usually just dealing uni-dimensionally. The nature of the conflict and the way it plays out will tend to be complex because it involves issues belonging to various dimensions. Each dimension presents a different type of challenge. Whereas Dimension 1 involves the willingness and ability to put oneself in the shoes of the other, looking at the world from their point of view, Dimension 2 perhaps involves a different kind of recognition of otherness – the generosity of spirit to see that other people might be 'serving other gods'. Letting in the possibility of these other gods can be challenging and surprisingly painful. In other respects Dimension 3 is perhaps the hardest because it is very hard to convey how life looks from more 'integral' states of awareness and consciousness.

Differentiating between these three 'dimensions' will not, of course, solve the deep and entrenched conflicts which affect human relationships. But this does offer a diagnostic tool so that we do not confuse issues of process and issues of 'self'. Similarly, we should not confuse issues of 'self' with those of ego development. By estimating what belongs where can at least avoid particular confusions and help find specific strategies that address the question of difference.

References

Darley, G and McKie, D, *Ian Nairn Words in Place*, Five Leaves, 2013

Cowan, C and Beck, D, *Spiral Dynamics*, Blackwell Business, 1996

Ferrer, J, *Revisioning Transpersonal Theory,* SUNY, 2002

Gadamer, H, *Truth and Method*, Continuum, 2004

Hillman, J, *The Soul's Code*, Warner, 1996

Kegan, R, *The Evolving Self*, Harvard University Press,1982

Lawley, J and Tompkins, P, Metaphors in Mind, The Developing Company, 2000

Pullman, P, *Northern Lights*, Scholastic Books, 1995

Rosenberg, M, *Nonviolent Communication*, Encinitas: Puddledancer, 2003

Said, E, *Orientalism*, Routledge & Kegan Paul, 1978

Wilber, K, *Integral Spirituality,* Integral Books, 2006

Aware Parenting

Marion Rose

I am so grateful that I trained as a psychosynthesis psychotherapist before I became a parent. The understandings I gained about my own experiences, combined with the knowledge about personality development from a psychospiritual perspective, have been deeply helpful in my parenting journey. My children are now 12 and 8 years old.

I had several threads to weave together when I became a parent: developmental psychology, psychosynthesis psychotherapy, and Aware Parenting. In this article, I will talk about Aware Parenting, which is congruent with a psychospiritual perspective.

I discovered Aware Parenting (www.awareparenting.com) whilst I was pregnant, and started to read Aletha Solter's books. Here I found the practical application of all I had learnt in developmental psychology and psychosynthesis, with an added extra. That extra piece was the understanding that babies are born with the ability to heal from daily stresses, as well as any traumas, that they experience. They don't need to wait until adulthood to go into therapy to heal from the painful experiences in their childhood; they can heal from birth onwards.

How does this healing happen? You won't be surprised to hear that one of the mechanisms is through crying. Babies cry for two reasons; to indicate an immediate need, and also to release stress and trauma from their bodies. However, in order for the crying to be healing, a baby needs to be held in the loving arms of someone who is present and empathic.

Some of the stresses and traumas babies experience include: stress in utero; traumatic birth; separation after birth; developmental frustrations; over stimulation; and frightening events. From this perspective, all babies experience uncomfortable feelings quite frequently, however aware we aim to be as parents.

Differentiating between crying to express an immediate need, and crying to release painful feelings, is quite a practice, particularly for most of us who were not held and listened to when we were upset as babies.

One of the main confusions for parents is to differentiate between hunger and painful feelings. However, there are very clear cues and communications from babies about whether they are hungry, or are simply feeling painful feelings that need to be heard. Another common confusion is between tiredness and a need to release feelings. In most other parenting paradigms, when a baby cries in the evening, it is assumed that the crying is caused by tiredness being uncomfortable, and that we need to stop the crying and get the baby to sleep.

However, in Aware Parenting, there is an understanding of the mechanisms of repression and dissociation. Babies (like children and adults) are less able to repress feelings when they are tired. So, before sleep, and particularly at the end of another day of new experiences, babies naturally cry to release tensions from their bodies. If we understand this process, and simply hold our baby, being present, listening to the feelings, telling her we are here with her, she will cry, and cry some more, and release all the feelings from the day. If we follow this process, we can notice certain things in the baby. Once she has expressed her feelings, she makes eye contact, she is relaxed in her body, she moulds into our hold, and she sleeps easily. From a psychospiritual perspective, babies return to Self during sleep; the more they are able to release the stresses of the day, the more easily they can return to their source during sleep.

However, because most people do not understand that crying is a natural healing mechanism, we tend to assume one of two things, depending on our parenting beliefs. The first is that that all crying indicates an unmet need, so we need to do something to prevent the crying. The second is that babies need to become independent early, so they need to learn to self-soothe. In the first case, the parent stops the feelings. In the second case, the baby learns to stop the feelings.

In the first case, there are a number of ways to stop the crying, generally using the parent's body:

1 Feeding for comfort
2 Movement – such as jiggling or rocking, or moving in a sling
3 Distraction – such as singing, or showing toys

In the second case, the ways are usually using things other than the parent's body:

1 Bottle feeding or feeding solids; or giving a dummy
2 Movement in a pram or in the car
3 Distraction – e.g. leaving the baby in a rocking cradle
4 Leaving the baby alone to cry

However, what all of these methods do, along with thumb-sucking, or clutching on to a toy or a blanket, is to create a state of dissociation. We can see this because of the look in the baby's eyes, which will be 'spaced-out', with an avoidance of eye contact.

Very quickly, a baby learns these habitual ways to disconnect from his feelings. The dissociated feelings accumulate in the body. This accumulation can be seen in many different ways. The baby starts to avoid eye contact, because eye contact connects him with his feelings, which he has learnt to avoid. He will start to smile less often, because disconnecting from his uncomfortable feelings means he needs to disconnect from his happier feelings too (as indicated on the Egg Diagram). He starts to feel agitated in his body – which can be felt as muscle tension, movement during sleep and an inability to concentrate for long. He starts to wake up more frequently, even though he is older and is physiologically able to sleep longer, simply because the feelings keep waking him up to be released.

He will also seem to need whatever it is we do to him to stop the feelings, more and more. So, a baby fed when he is upset will seem to need feeding more and more frequently, even though his tummy is bigger and can hold more milk. A baby who is rocked to sleep will need a longer period of rocking to get to sleep.

A baby who has a dummy or clutches on to a soft toy or blanket will do that more and more often and for longer periods. A baby who sucks his thumb or fingers will also do this more often and for longer periods of time. A baby who is distracted will seem to need to be played with all the time. Aware Parenting calls these mechanisms of dissociation Control Patterns, a concept which is congruent with psychosynthesis teaching on addiction and abuse. When a baby experiences stress or trauma, and the resultant feelings are not listened to or released, she needs to do something to stop herself from feeling the feelings. The more severe the trauma, the more extreme the control patterns need to be.

These control patterns change in form throughout a person's life, if the feelings underlying them are not felt and expressed. For example, a baby may be rocked when he is upset, and will then learn to move when he is upset. He might become a child who can 'never sit still' and an adult who is always busy. A baby who sucks her thumb when she is upset might become a nail-biter as a child and a smoker as a teenager. A baby who is fed when upset might become a child who eats when unhappy and an adult who drinks coffee or alcohol when facing uncomfortable feelings.

All babies are seen as, at their core, aware, present, able to concentrate, wanting to connect, cooperate and contribute. When a baby is showing behaviours that indicate an accumulation of uncomfortable feelings (e.g. avoiding eye contact, being agitated, or thumb-sucking), she is less connected with herself. When she is given plenty of opportunity to express and release pent-up feelings through crying in the loving arms of a parent, she returns to a natural state of calm, relaxed presence. She makes eye contact, she is relaxed, she sleeps easily. She is more who she really is. From a psychospiritual perspective, as her personality structures develop, she is more connected with her Self. Her 'I' becomes a more accurate reflection of her true Self.

This Aware Parenting paradigm continues throughout childhood. Most of the behaviours that parents find challenging – children hitting, biting, not cooperating, not listening, doing things that they know that the parents don't want, not sleeping, swearing, throwing things – all these often also indicate pent-up feelings.

So, instead of resorting to punishments or rewards, from this approach we see that the child simply needs connection plus release. Connection is vital. Tears and tantrums release feelings such as sadness, frustration, confusion, grief, and overwhelm from the body. Laughter releases feelings such as fear, anxiety, frustration, helplessness and powerlessness.

Children rarely come to us and ask us if we will hold them whilst they cry. Their requests come in code – in all those behaviours listed above, and more. When they call out in these coded ways, we can go in and connect with various tools – including connection, connection plus loving limits, and connection plus attachment play. These strategies help the child release feelings through laughter or crying with connection. When the child has released the relevant chunk of feelings, the troublesome behaviour goes away. This is because we have dispersed the root cause of the behaviour.

So, Aware Parenting is congruent with a psychospiritual approach – it sees that at core, children naturally all have qualities, such as connection, cooperation and contribution, and when they are behaving in ways that aren't expressing these qualities they simply need connection plus release.

Another gift of this kind of parenting is that the development of the super-ego is affected. Without punishments, shaming, 'shoulds' and so on, children stay more deeply connected with their true motivations to make life more wonderful for others. In fact, this model questions the traditional models of moral development, which is based upon studying children exposed to parenting paradigms that use punishments and rewards, shaming and 'shoulding'.

Even very young children can be gentle with other children and pets, and can be happy to share, and to listen and cooperate. These are qualities we are all born with, and which we can stay connected with if we are given plenty of opportunity to cry and laugh with loving support.

One of the main benefits of Aware Parenting for the child is that the more of her feelings that are listened to and accepted, the less she needs to split off from. The more can be integrated into her sense of self, and the more of a sense of unconditional love she receives. The more feelings that her parents are able to be present within themselves, the more they will be able to hear, mirror and allow to be released in her. The more her personality will develop as a relatively accurate reflection of her Self.

Aware Parenting gives us practical tools to parent within a psychospiritual context. It is also an approach that is relevant to us as adults. For example, it gives us a way of understanding how and when we dissociate from our feelings, such as by repetitive use of Facebook, eating chocolate, tidying the house or exercising obsessively. It helps us understand the genesis of our control patterns; for example, we may remember that we used to clutch on to a soft toy as a baby, then avoided having friends as a child and intimacy with our partners as an adult. Or perhaps we used to pick our nose as a child, pick our spots as a teenager and pick on others as an adult. We can also recognise that our ways of dealing with our own feelings affect how we interpret our baby or child's behaviour. For example, if we tend to eat when we are upset, when our baby cries we are likely to interpret that she is hungry, and will feed her. In that way, she learns to interpret her own inner feeling experience as hunger and will ask to eat when she is upset. If we tend to distract ourselves with the Internet when we are upset, we are likely to think our baby needs distracting when she is upset and so will distract her with games and toys, and then she learns to do the same.

Sitting with a baby crying in our arms, knowing that all of his needs are met, is a powerful experience. In order to listen to his feelings, we need to be willing to hear the cries of our own baby self. The baby in us that was left alone to cry or the baby in us that was always distracted from our feelings. The more we are able to listen to our own feelings from when we were a baby, the more we can listen to his feelings – of overwhelm, confusion, fear, sadness, mourning, helplessness, frustration and so on. Sitting with our baby in our arms as he cries, through a whole cycle of crying, we may find ourselves thinking of his birth or of a time during the pregnancy or when we argued with our partner when he was a small baby. Our intuition may tell us what he is releasing and expressing. At the end of this expressing, if he has completed releasing a whole chunk of feelings, he will return to a state of calm present awareness.

In the many hundreds of times I have been with my children through these experiences, and the many times I have been present with parents and their babies, I have witnessed the baby, once he naturally finishes crying, entering a particular state of presence. He makes eye contact. He is incredibly calm and relaxed yet alert. A quality of deep peace comes into the room, such as one might experience on a meditation retreat. The little one looks like a Buddha, although of course we know that he is one with Self without being conscious of this. His body is relaxed, free from tension, and he is free to sleep easily.

Similarly, children will cry or tantrum to express painful feelings. There are a number of ways that the crying can start. One way is when a small event starts off a big reaction. Here, the child is using the small event as a pretext to release bigger feelings. She cries when the last biscuit is broken, or when her favourite t-shirt is in the washing machine. As we become familiar with the release process, at these times we can avoid fixing things, and simply be present and empathic with her as she cries. A baby needs to be held to feel safe when she cries. A child, once mobile, does not always need to be held in our arms, but she does need to be held in our loving awareness. Once she has had a big cry, we often find that she won't really mind about the last biscuit or the favourite t-shirt, since that was only a pretext for the crying.

In Aware Parenting, for laughter or crying to be healing, we need what is called the balance of attention. The balance is between emotional safety on the one hand

and the stimulus for the feelings on the other. At the exact sweet spot, somewhere between these two, the feelings are expressed most intensely.

Another way is a 'loving limit'. A loving limit is the balance of attention in operation. A loving limit contains no harshness, no punishment or disconnection. Its purpose is simply to help the child express and release the feelings that were underlying the challenging behaviour, so that the behaviour, which was only a symptom, then stops. If we try to stop the behaviour without listening to the underlying feelings, the behaviour will simply return, or show up in a different form. Loving limits pair empathy with a limit. (This is the balance of attention – the emotional safety with the stimulus for the feelings). If the situation is urgent, for example the child is about to hurt someone or something, we start with the limit (ideally in a calm, loving, centred tone); "I won't let you hit me", and pair it with the empathy, "I see that you are upset". When we find the exact balance of attention, and if the child feels enough emotional safety in general, the child will then cry, rage, or tantrum. These were the feelings driving the acting out behaviour. The child doesn't want to hurt anyone; she simply wasn't feeling safe in the moment to drop into the tears and tantrums.

If the situation is less urgent, we can start with the empathy, and then add the limit, for example, "I see that you really want to watch something on the iPad and I'm not willing for you to watch anything more now. I'm here and I'm listening. Yes, you really love watching things, and I'm not willing for you to watch anymore..." It is the combination of the two that create the sweet spot, for the healing tears to come.

In this way, we can avoid either being permissive or authoritarian as parents. We can practice democratic discipline, which is all about finding ways for everyone's needs to get met. We can and search for the underlying causes of challenging behaviour (in ourselves as well as our children). We can help them (and us) express and release feelings in an empathic environment, thus creating connection and harmony.

For me, Aware Parenting is an approach which combines the most up-to-date research on child development and psychotherapy, into a very practical approach for parents. It includes particular ways of understanding babies and children, and precise tools which help a child flourish whilst staying connected with her authentic self. Of course, because most of us still have our own blind spots and have more psychological work to do, our children will still carry some repressed and dissociated parts, some control patterns, and some disconnection from themselves and others, yet much less than what we have carried.

And so, evolution occurs, with each generation carrying fewer psychological burdens, whilst being more deeply connected to the joy, presence and love that we innately are.

Bibliography

Solter, A, *Helping Young Children Flourish*, Shining Star Press, 1989

Solter, A, *Tears and Tantrums: What To Do When Babies and Children Cry*, Shining Star Press, 1998

Solter, A, *The Aware Baby*, revised edition, Shining Star Press, 2001

Solter, A, *Raising Drug-Free Kids: 100 Tips for Parents*, Da Capo Press, 2006

Solter, A, *Attachment Play: How to Solve Children's Behaviour Problems with Play, Laughter and Connection*, Shining Star Press, 2013

Love Transforms

Veronique Maria

When someone asks me how, with all my history, I've became so solid, articulate and comfortable in my own skin, I'm baffled. Then I tell them it was Psychosynthesis; eighteen years of weekly psychotherapy, eight years of a professional training and several years writing papers, poems and prose describing my experiences. It's difficult to put my finger on it exactly 'what Psychosynthesis is to me'. Psychosynthesis helped me grow from a shy, inarticulate girl, into a strong, self-assured woman.

I tell people Psychosynthesis helped me build a house inside of myself...

In 2013 I was awarded a three month Artist's Residency by the Wurlitzer Foundation USA. They provided me with an old adobe casita on seventeen acres of woodland in New Mexico and invited me to 'do my creative thing'. Thousands of miles from home, family and friends, and with no car, phone or internet, I found myself 'listening' to myself, others and the environment with new, and expanded levels of heightened awareness.

I'd originally intended to use my time in Taos to write a film script and work on video. It soon became clear this residency was about exploring who I am when there's no project and my layers are peeled right back. 8,000 feet up a sacred mountain, with limited oxygen, I felt permanently high. Stripped bear, each moment had a quality of prayer.

In 'normal' life back home in England I'd been striving to surrender to the unknown but fear often held me back. Trust seemed easier in Taos. Soon after arriving, I purchased four beautifully illustrated story books, one of which was Thomas Blue Eagle's Ledger Book. These were the first gifts I'd ever dared buy for my much hoped for grandchild. Not willing to give up on that dream, I returned to my casita and wrote the following poem.

Thomas Blue Eagle's Ledger Book

I bought
b o o k s
for you today.
four precious symbols
of my desire to dream you
into being.

I've been dreaming of you for years,
and I think of you almost everyday now
I wonder when you will come to me
I want to make you blankets and shawls and tiny booties
I want to gather you up in my arms – tell you mama will always love you

I want to sew with you, dance with you and lay down and stroke you

I want you to have everything a child should have
and be protected from all that children shouldn't have to bear

I wonder when you will come to me

I am dreaming you darling,
and daydreaming you
into being
with all
m y
love.

A month later, when my son announced the conception of his daughter, I was in heaven, awe and wonder. I celebrated with gratitude and rituals.

Many of my experiences in New Mexico were monumental. Never knowing what's coming next, I wrote the following:

Blessed Art Thou…

Dawn, New Mexico 2014

Dogs

Wild dogs searching for truth came sniffing in my casita.
Hairy mongrels with wet noses and wagging tails.

I tried to catch them as they danced around the house.
Jumping up onto my bed many times and then hiding in dark corners.

They had twinkles in their eyes and sometimes their tales swept the floor.

Therapy 2014

"I'll be fifty five at the end of this month."

Pause.

"I trained extensively as an artist, a psychotherapist, and an applied psychosynthesis practitioner. For what? Pivoting between fifty and sixty I'm out on a high wire. Not a comfortable place."

"What would be comfortable?"

"When I reflect back over my life, I remember how I thought it was going to be, especially in my mid teens, when I had a really strong sense of who I was and where I was going. It didn't turn out quite as I thought it would. I often wonder what I could have done differently."

Pause.

"Mmmm comfortable? I suppose that would be when I am really settled and everything seems right. Actually I get that feeling quite a lot. I'm not talking about that sort of 'comfortable' though, I'm talking about being comfortable about being mortal – a deep sense of comfort.
Maybe the comfort I'm talking about is born out of being on track, aligned with one's life purpose, at peace with life and death and able to hold one's self steady in any situation.

I remember feeling fully in my body when I was fifteen. That feeling of vibrancy, determination, strength and vitality; a sense nothing could stop me from having life. I was focused and in love. If I had died in that moment I imagine I might have felt whole and complete.

I remember prancing across Hampstead Heath enjoying nature and my body as if they were one.

I was wearing my grandpa's bola hat with a peacock feather in it. My sixties blouse stitched from beautiful soft green material, hung loosely over my young skin. Black tailored trousers sat comfortably secure around my waist. Everything was exactly as it should be. The present moment was divine. The future planned, clear and tangible. My memory of that moment returns to me often. My sense of it is so strong."

Dusk, Sussex Hospital 1989

With my face pushed up against gloss painted plaster work on the ceiling, I watched my body thirty feet below me, in the hospital bed. Everyone looked small. Medics busied themselves around 'me' down there whilst I occupied myself with ceiling textures. I was calm and strangely, detached from critical activities below. Seemingly suspended in space, neither occupying my body nor the ether, the building's architecture seemed to be acting as some kind of a boundary for me. Occasionally I wondered whether I might be able to slip through the ceiling but I seemed to be hesitating or resisting that next move. I wasn't afraid, I just didn't know what I would be going into.

Then, suddenly I seemed to make a clear choice and returned to my body. The nurse greeted me warmly. I could see relief and delight in her face. 'Hello. Welcome back. I thought for a moment we had lost you."

Apparently I had been trying to sit up in the bed when I suddenly felt dizzy, and couldn't breathe. (I re-membered that that had happening just before I went to the ceiling.) 'Your skin colour turned grey and you started to disappear. We called the crash team. We thought you were going'.

Therapy 2007

"I'd been planning to go to art college since I was about ten. I believed whole heartedly, the life I dreamt of would materialise after school. My love would come with me. I knew every inch of her body just as well as I knew my own. I knew the way she breathed, and the way we breathed together, the way her chest rose when I touched her and how to stroke her to make her shudder. I loved the way her chest bones sat proud and how down covered her jaw. I knew how her blonde locks would fall over her face when we laid together. I understood things she couldn't talk about, and I knew that I loved her. Her vibration was divine. Nothing could change my devotion to her and us, nothing that is, except for her."

Taos Mountain 2014

Breathing Heart

I went out
looking for you today,
and
found you in the Indian land briefly.

My heart opened wide
and suddenly,
It felt unexpected and ancient.

In the gentle silence
and the vast open space,
my heart became like lungs,

Eagles' wings spread out within my chest

and I could breathe,
speak truths,
and know

all
there is
to know.

Or at least that is how it felt in that moment.

I found you today in the open plains,
in the mountain and in the sky.

It was as if you came to me
and
showed me all I need to know

You came to me today
and then briefly
like lovers in a moment of communion, we were one.

Tate Modern, London 2049

Scene 1:

Millennium Bridge, Thames London.

Small family group walk from St Paul's Cathedral to Tate Modern.

They look up at neon lights on building.

Group approaches gallery doors.

Whispering voices 'blessed art thou'.

Sounds build up, layered into chants.

Noise of Turbines mingle with chants - 'Blessed Art thou'.

Artist looks outside window up towards moon.

She shivers.

Turns head downwards.

Cold pavement level - woman, curled up alone, keeps from freezing.

Strawberry Tree, Sussex UK 2008

Scene 2:

Garden studio: large timber log cabin.

Natural light streaming in.

Ceiling vaulted.

Roof windows.

Sky views.

Artist VM aged 40 making performance art.

Sweeping pulverised Paw Paw fruit across timber floor boards.

Orange flesh/black seeds mingle with yellow fruit skin.

Some pulp caught in grooves of painted pine floor.

VM sweeps pulp into a pile using long handled broom.

Friend drumming gently - sits in corner of room.

Video camera in corner on tripod records events.

Moonlight, Surrey Hills, 2004

come to me

I
have
b e e n
w a i t i n g
d r e a m i n g
longing for you
the ache of desire – the wanting
for years – possibly lifetimes
heavy with anticipation
ancient searching – praying for your touch
tonight the moon knows, hanging large, heavy, low
I can see you – feel you – delight in you
full with warm pink peach
you are in my being
with painful longing
and
in every moment that I dare reach out for you
agony ecstasy
you are my fire and I burn for you
there is no lover like this...................but this one
eternal internal universal
dark night skies, deep oceans,
r i c h v e l v e t
b l a c k
sophisticated
m a t u r e
r a w
come
to
me

Therapy 2009

"I hadn't expected that in letting her hold my heart in her hands I had somehow given her the power to change my vision. I am broken hearted. Everything around me is crashing and changing."

"Same as your first love. Can you feel the reverberations?"

"Yes. Love keeps re-forming itself. The revised form still revolves around creativity and art, (which is a relief!) but it is complex and often effected by lovers."

Therapy 2012

"Death terrifies me. I tell myself it's okay but when it comes close, I'm terrified. Flying in an aeroplane, having an anaesthetic, surgery, that kind of thing. Then the cancer scare of course! I never felt so afraid and alone.

Plus I can't bear to break attachments either. It's always the horizontal pull which affects my relationship with death I suppose.

Out of body experiences remind me there's no death only transformation to another form, but when push comes to shove it's so hard to remember that. I seem so unable to surrender a lot of the time. My body is tense, braced for disasters which are probably unlikely to ever happen.

When I'm skiing, and I'm on top of a mountain looking down at the sheer drop below, sometimes I freeze up. Standing there considering what to do, the more I think about it the more I resist movement. I imagine terrible things happening: accident, injury, pain, death. I think, if I just stay here (stuck!) I'll be safe. So I stay a little longer till I realise I am only just 'alive' here, not fully living.

I don't exactly know what happens to make the shift, but somehow I find something within myself and I'm able to let go of the fear, surrender to the unknown, lean my body forwards down into the sheer drop in front of me and allow the rest of my body to follow.

As I'm falling towards the void I say to myself, 'keep going, keep leaning forwards, keep surrendering'. It's empowering. I feel held by something far greater than me, a universal power, a higher self, who knows?

When I feel stuck in my life I try to remember skiing processes to manage fear."

Therapy 2014

"I keep thinking of the words 'Blessed Art thou'. What makes anyone blessed? My mother told me she doesn't like me, has no desire to see me, apparently I am the only person in the world she cannot get along with. How can anyone feel 'blessed' when their own mother says that?"

Therapy 2000

Geoff phoned asking me to visit as soon as possible. "Amanda would really like to see you." I knew she was ill. She'd been ill almost twelve years. We'd spent more days talking about her health than I cared to remember. I always thought she'd pull through. I hadn't quite clocked the urgency. I went straight away though.

Geoff had gone to collect Laura their daughter, from the airport. She'd been sent away to Italy for a trip. She'd hardly arrived there when they called her back home urgently. Amanda was deteriorating rapidly. No one had expected it to be this fast. Had we all been in colluding in hope?

I went upstairs to the single bedroom she'd moved to when she knew she'd be having visitors and nursing support. She'd painted it pale aqua and hung images of angels all around her. She was like a bag of bones. I'd just seen her on Sunday. She'd asked me to pop in with lettuces. She'd come to the door, vibrant and appreciative as ever. If I had known then that her time was ticking away so fast I would have accepted her offer to come in but I had no idea. I believed she was fighting this thing and my new lover was about to leave for India the next day so I had made her my priority, as we had needed time to say our goodbyes.

I went upstairs. Amanda's brother was downstairs with a couple of friends. I sat very close to Amanda's bedside and held her hand. She said, "I keep slipping away, coming and going, I don't know where I am." She seemed confused and troubled. I didn't know what to say. Is this what happens when we leave here go to the other side? Do we travel back and forth until we're ready to let go?

I wanted to ask her what it was like there, on the other side, but it didn't seem appropriate. I was shocked at her appearance and concerned for her distress. Urgency was all around. I was sitting at death's door with my dearest friend.

Originally my art college tutor, Amanda had inspired and encouraged me with incredible passion. Being of similar age and both with children, we soon became good friends. "You're here with me now. Try not to worry." I said. It seemed stupid though. I felt as if I was on a train about to leave the station and in a moment I would have to jump off and let Amanda do the rest of the journey on her own. I was unprepared. I didn't know how to be.

We held hands as she settled a bit, "Yes I'm here now" she said, slightly relieved, but after that she kept slipping away before the end of her sentences. "It's as if I'm falling backwards falling away."

And then she grasped hold of my hand as if she wanted to say something really important. She was using all of her energy to collect herself together.

She said, "I love your work, I really love it, I think it's amazing." Then she slipped away completely. Those were her last words to me.

Cathedral, West Sussex 2000

Scene 3:

VM lying belly down on flagstone floor - centre of the cathedral isle.

Arms out. Legs slightly apart. Appears frozen.

Hands flat on floor above her head.

In front of VM - Traditional light wood coffin raised on trestle stand.

Flowers draped over closed coffin lid.

Fresh white lilies, ferns, fall over casket sides.

Side chapel - woman praying.

Head bowed over hands.

Rosary beads woven through fingers.

Chanting "blessed art thou and blessed is the fruit of thy womb"

VM pushes her face deeper into stone.

Spring 2014

Love Poem

The more places I go, the more things I do,
The more people I meet, the more I miss you.
Grief is a peculiar thing.
The thread between us remains even when everything else seems to have peeled away.
In fact without all the clutter I am much more aware of it.

In the end,
when all the stuff of life is gone,
When all the complications and confusions have melted and the fibres are dry,
We will stand apart like tall stringed instruments
Golden threads revealed, stretching across the universe
unbreakable
eternal
love

Summer 2049

Scene 4:

River Thames near St Paul's Cathedral.

Family Group prepare to walk over Millennium bridge.

Elderly woman VM (90s) to granddaughter (34):

"I wanted so much to make a difference. I devoted my life to art. Do you think that anything has changed? Do you think we understand the importance and value of self and collective expression any better now? Do you think we are more in touch with the moment, the materials, the making? Have we repositioned art and artist into the centre of our society and value system?" "I don't know grandma. What I do know is that you have had and do have a massive impact on the people who see your work and hear you speak about art. You touch them deeply. I have seen it for myself time and time again. People cry, get down on their knees, get exhilarated and animated, you bring on all sorts of significant and valuable responses grandma. Let's go see the show right now and do the press thing. I am so excited for you."

Son (70s) holds elderly woman's hand tenderly. Helps her into wheel chair.

"Darling you are the best and most important thing I ever created in my entire life. We made you from pure love you know." She touches his face and smiles deeply. He receives her touch and grins lovingly.

Pregnant granddaughter (28) carefully tucks shawl around grandmas legs, checks feet on foot rests. Gently pushes chair across bridge to Tate.

Gallery Entrance - assistant introduces group to awaiting guests.

Group walks into gallery.

Press awaits.

Curator says:

"Welcome everyone, to 'Blessed Art...' Thank you for coming along to the Tate today. We are so pleased you are here and hope you will enjoy the tour. I am delighted to see so many faces. To those who don't already know me I am Isabella Cairns, exhibitions director here at the Tate Modern and directing curator for this exhibition. I'm really very excited to show you this exhibition - a major retrospective spanning 1974 and 2049 by Veronique Maria. We will take you through the exhibition shortly. Ms Maria will give personal insights into some of the ideas, processes and intensions behind her work. The show is deliberately not laid out chronologically. The intention is for you to experience the exhibition as a whole life's work and to see and sense the work of one woman's intimate life rather than a linear developmental process. We will mention significant mentors and inspiration as we go alone. If you have questions please feel free to ask at any point."

Autumn 2002 Therapy

"When people have blessed me in life, especially those whom I respect and admire, I have felt like a brand new sail boat being launched from its slipway with expensive champagne.

I've felt incredibly affirmed and been much more able to move forwards with confidence and power as a consequence of these blessings."

"Who has affirmed you in this way?"

"Many; my grandparents are the obvious ones, the constant ones. My mother encouraged my creativity when I was young when she let me paint of my bedroom wall, and then later it was people in the Psychosynthesis training and artists I respect. Awards, prizes and being patronised is affirming too of course, and friends, audiences, and lovers are very significant as well. Most of those affirmations seem to be related to my authenticity, creativity and courage as an artist though. Is that what you meant?"

"And what about your first love, your first lover?"

"Well she has always admired me on some level and rejected me on another of course. She mirrors my familiar experience. Constantly affirming grandparents and persistently rejecting mother rolled into one. It's complicated to live with such extreme poles – externalised and then internalised.

You always bring her back into the conversation. Do you think there is something unresolved there for me? You always challenge me to look inside the dark dusty corners that I might otherwise prefer to ignore!"

Autumn 1987

Scene 5:
Hospital Theatre.
Male surgeon cuts woman's naked belly horizontally.
Passes scalpel to theatre sister.
His hands enter deep inside wound.
Beside operating table sits cheap plastic bucket.
Inside bucket - Womb lies in blood.
Surgeon drops second (unknown) organ into bucket.
Blood splashes up bucket sides.
Drops spill on handle.
Organ hits womb, falls in beside it - slips in comfortably.
New camera shot - questionable object in bucket - Foetus?
Other end of room:
Woman with wild flower bouquet slowly places individual stalks carefully into another bucket.
Takes time positioning/arranging flowers/foliage.
Another corner of operating theatre.
VM pours remains of Paw Paw fruit (brushed from studio floor) into third bucket.
Paw Paw slips into bucket.
VM repeats "blessed art thou, blessed is the fruit of thy womb..."

Winter 2007

"How was it for you to be with your first lover again this weekend?"

"She is gorgeous. I love her deeply and am inspired at how our love has transformed."

Winter, Many Moments Over Several Decades – Merging (1958-2049)

```
Scene 6:
Visceral Scene.
Hospital.
Layers of images - bodies, life, death, collecting things in buckets, gathering, sweeping.
Drum keeps playing.
Same scenes are being projected as video installation onto massive wall Tate gallery.
Press/journalist and others audience members observe.
```

Winter 2010

"Why is she more prominent than other loves?

Does she lead you back to my mother? As my first love? In an ideal world?"

Winter 1998

```
Scene 7:
Lush English Garden.
Overgrown, semi tropical.
VM making prayer beads whispering 'blessed art thou'.
Tiny clay balls, moulded in her fingers, fall into a metal pot – 'tink'.
```

Winter 2009

"She is not my original love…my art is my all time lover. She is constant and transforms all other loves into new forms. She saves me, holds me, never gives up on me…

I am able to take more risks in life because I have this lover who holds, enables and guides me."

Spring 2009

Scene 8:
Garden Sussex.
Late Spring.
Mid Day.
Secluded, slightly over grown Sussex garden.
Warm sunny day.
VM (50) wearing loosely fitting clothing.
Thin cotton sun dress falls around her shoulders.
She has bare feet and is nearly naked.
Dry grass runs through her toes.
Her finger tips tickle seeds pods and flowers as she passes.
The air is still.
A grass snake slithers through a patch of damp earth between compost heap and pond.
She walks inside the house and becomes much older...(99)

2059

Light modern house full of texture, colour, care.
Eclectic mix of mid century and faded style.
VM sits down at table strew with love poems/photographs.
VM takes an old A4 email from forty six years earlier.
Puts on glasses.

Reads silently: "I need to go slowly. I am afraid. You seem too good to be true. M :) x". "Lean in to me and trust sweetheart, all we can do is trust and keep communicating. V xxx".

M (97) enters room.

Sits close beside VM.

Slips loving hands around VM.

Leans over and kisses VM's neck.

VM turns to M and says "We learnt to ride over the ocean darling, we have been very blessed.

M "Yes my darling we have been very blessed."

VM takes M's face in her hands and says "Blessed art thou".

M touches VM tenderly. Pulls VM close to her and says:

"Yes my beautiful, and blessed is our fruit."

Spring 2013 – Wondrous Life (Still Moment from a Video)

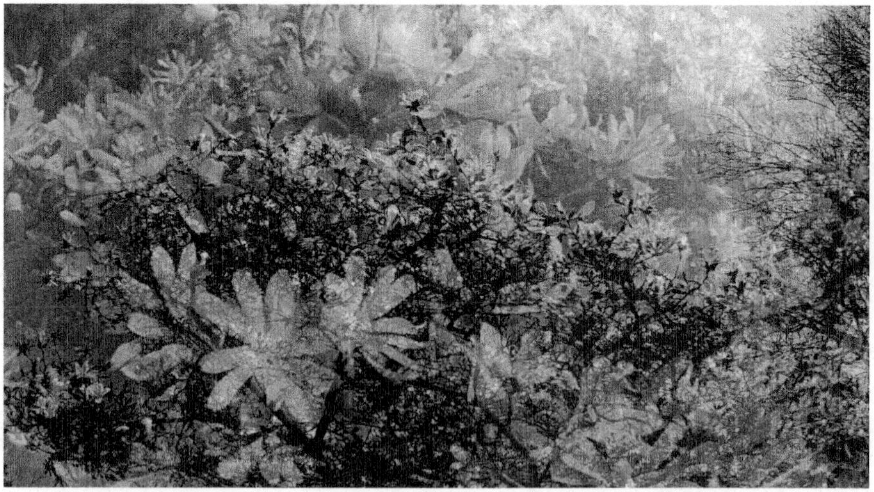

Author Biographies

JARLATH F BENSON BA, DipSoc, MSocSc, MMedSc, trained as a Social Worker, studied psychosynthesis at the Irish Institute of Psychosynthesis, subsequently qualified as a psychoanalytic psychotherapist (Belfast) and later qualified as a Group Analyst (Dublin). He has been a long time faculty member at the Institute of Psychosynthesis London. Jarlath was formerly chairman of the Northern Ireland Institute of Human relations and then its director from 1996-1999. He is on the advisory board of the Irish Institute of Psychosocial Studies and is a member of the Irish Psychoanalytical Association. His textbook *Working More Creatively with Groups* is in its third edition and he has published a number of papers and chapters on the psychological aspects of the Northern Ireland conflict.

KRISTINA BRODE PhD in Education (field of Clinical Psychology), has worked as a Psycho-oncologist since 1984 and developed and evaluated Systemic Cancer Care Program (SYSPEP®). She was involved in several projects at Tumorcenters, (Berlin 2005-2009) and Head of Circadian Institute for Applied Psychosynthesis, near Cologne (1984-2002). She is a Trainer and Coach in various organisations (Siemens, Caritas, German Telecom). The work she loves most is Archetypal Psychosynthesis, working with Mythology.

DERYN COPPER PhD in Psychology (Auck), MA (Hons), Dip Tchg, Diplomas in Psychosynthesis Counselling and Psychosynthesis Psychotherapy (NZ), MNZAC, Post-Grad. Cert in Professional Supervision, is Co-chair of PAnzA, teaches ethics in the Dip Counselling and Dip Psychotherapy programmes for the Institute of Psychosynthesis NZ and has a private practice in Auckland.

JESS CURTIS trained to be a teacher at the Central School of Speech and Drama, and later acquired an LGSM at the Guildhall school of Music. In 2002 she completed the therapeutic counselling course at the Institute of Psychosynthesis, and not being offered a place on the MA course there, she moved on to study and graduate from the Psychosynthesis and Education Trust in 2009. Her MA Dissertation title was *Sound in the Therapy Room*. A later study of EFT (Energy Freedom Technique) has contributed to her ongoing involvement and therapeutic work with energy as vibration.

THEO DIJKMAN MA is a psychotherapist and supervisor working in private practice and a faculty member of the Institute of Psychosynthesis. He has over 20 years experience of working in senior management positions in mental health in the voluntary sector and continues to deliver training to staff and management teams as a consultant. Originally from the Netherlands, Theo has brought up his family in Scotland where he loves the hills and wide open spaces.

JOAN EVANS MA in Psychosynthesis Psychotherapy is co-founder and director of the Institute of Psychosynthesis, responsible for designing its academic and training programmes and editing a Textbook for Training in Psychosynthesis. She has trained practitioners in the UK and Europe for 40 years, helping to steer counselling and psychotherapy training towards attaining professional status. She was the first chair of the European Federation for Psychosynthesis Psychotherapy, Chair of HIPS and a member of the Governing Board of the UKCP (1995-99).

ROGER EVANS is a psychospiritual psychotherapist registered with the UKCP. He is also a Co-Founder and a Director with his wife Joan, of the Institute of Psychosynthesis, London, where he is currently a senior faculty member, specialising in working with the Self as a spiritual context to understand individual and group psychological disturbances – specifically the nature of Spiritual Emergence and Emergency and how to work with these dilemmas. He is the managing partner of a Leadership Consultancy, CLC and has extensive international public and private sector consulting experience in Europe, Scandinavia, North America, the Middle East, India and Africa. He was a non-executive director of the board of the NHS Personnel Group, and served as a board member of the Technology Management School at Chalmers School of Technology and Management in Gothenberg, Sweden. He is the co-author with Peter Russell of the *The Creative Manager*, and is currently finishing a book on the dimensions of *Great Human Leadership*.

DOROTHY FIRMAN EdD is the president and director of The Synthesis Center, in Amherst, Massachusetts. She has been running psychosynthesis trainings for over thirty-five years. She is a licensed mental health counsellor, a Board Certified Coach and a Professor of Graduate Psychology, as well as being an author.

HARRY JENKINS MA in Psychosynthesis Psychotherapy, UKCP reg, BACP accredited. Harry works in private practice in the village of Penn, which lies between High Wycombe, Amersham and Beaconsfield, Bucks. Harry's work is enhanced by his deep interest in non-duality, a mystical spiritual path.

VERONIQUE MARIA has been working full time in the arts since 1970's. Working across disciplines (painting, sculpture, installation, live art performance, film, writing) 'body' is always central to her art practice. 1995-1998 she trained as a Psychosynthesis Psychotherapist and in 2003 she had graduated with a Masters where she Applied Psychosynthesis to her professional art practice. Supported by Arts Council England since 1994, and awarded numerous international residencies including New Mexico, Ireland and Iceland, Veronique exhibits/performs widely in places ranging from Tate Modern London, to the Volcano Museum Iceland, and a Cliff Edge With A Horse, West Cornwall. Her work is in public collections across the world including Iceland, Arizona, and UK. She has worked with artists such as Antony Gormley, Janine Antony and Danny Rolph.

JESSICA NELSON MA in Psychosynthesis Psychotherapy. Jessica is a faculty member and facilitator at the Institute of Psychosynthesis. Jessica practices as a psychotherapist in Buckinghamshire. She is married, with three young adult children, writes poetry and fiction, and is particularly interested in expressing her ever-deepening experience of Love in matter through the creative process.

JULIE O'BRIEN BA, Dip Psychosynthesis Counselling (NZ), Dip Psychosynthesis Psychotherapy (NZ), Associate Member PAnzA. After 15 years of clinical practice, Julie is taking a sabbatical from her psychotherapy and supervision private practice, and her teaching role at the Institute of Psychosynthesis NZ. Email: julie.obrien@xtra.co.nz.

WILL PARFITT has forty years experience of working with personal and spiritual development. Author, Kabbalah teacher, UKCP registered psychosynthesis psychotherapist and course leader, Will lives in Glastonbury offering psychotherapy, spiritual guidance and supervision plus well-established distance learning courses. Books by Will include: *The Complete Guide to the Kabbalah* (Rider, UK, 2001); *Psychosynthesis: The Elements and Beyond* (PSA, UK, 2006); *The Something and Nothing of Death* (PSA, UK, 2008); and *Psychosynthesis: New Perspectives* [editor] (PSA, UK, 2009). You can find more information on Will and his current work on his website: www.willparfitt.com.

JAY RAMSAY originally came to Psychosynthesis in his mid-20's, in the mid 1980's, when the Institute was at Cambridge Gate. He's the author of 35 books of poetry, non-fiction, and classic Chinese translation: most recently *Agistri Notebook* (KFS, 2014), *Monuments* (Waterloo Press, 2014), and *Shu Jing – the Book of History* (Penguin Classics, 2014). He's also poetry editor of *Caduceus* magazine, working in private practice as a UKCP accredited psychosynthesis psychotherapist and healer, also running personal development workshops. Website: www.jayramsay.co.uk

ROBYN ROGERS Diploma in Psychosynthesis Counselling (NZ), Diploma in Psychosynthesis Psychotherapy (NZ), Registered Psychotherapist MNZAC MPAnzA. Robyn has a private practice, teaches Fundamentals and Foundation Year programmes for the Institute of Psychosynthesis NZ, offers supervision, has developed and facilitated Treaty workshops throughout Aotearoa/NZ, is a court approved facilitator and offers supervision.

MARION ROSE BSc, PhD, DipCouns, DipPsych, FPCF FPCC, is a graduate of the Institute of Psychosynthesis and now lives and works in Australia. She is a Level Two Aware Parenting Instructor. Websites: www.marionrose.net, www.parentingwithpresence.net, awpsupport@iinet.net.au.

RICHARD SCHAUB PhD and BONNEY GULINO SCHAUB RN, MS are co-directors of the New York Psychosynthesis Institute. They teach psychospiritual

approaches to healthcare to business organizations, hospitals, treatment centres and schools. Their most recent book is The Florentine Promise.
Email: drrichardschaub@gmail.com.

ABBY SEIXAS is a psychotherapist, author and speaker specialising in issues of life balance. She offers workshops and retreats as well as her popular Deep River groups. Her work has been featured on national and local television, radio and print media, including NBCs *The Today Show, O, The Oprah Magazine, Self, Woman's Day* and *Body + Soul.* Abby studied psychosynthesis with Roberto Assagioli and has practiced psychosynthesis-oriented psychotherapy for thirty-five years. She has been a consultant and clinical trainer and supervisor at centres in the US and abroad, including England, the Netherlands and Russia. Websites: www.deepriv-erwithin.com and www.facebook.com/DeepRiverWithin, Email: abby@deepriv-erwithin.com.

KEITH SILVESTER trained at the Institute of Psychosynthesis, London, graduating as a psychotherapist in 1990. Between 2003 and 2010 he was Director of Programmes of the Psychosynthesis & Education Trust in London, where he continues to work as a supervisor and trainer. He has a private psychotherapy practice, is Chair of the Training Committee of the Humanistic & Integrative College of UKCP, and has recently qualified as a practitioner of the Alexander Technique.

STEVE SIMPSON is a Faculty Member, trainer and Senior Supervisor at the Institute of Psychosynthesis, London. He is in private practice as a psychosynthesis psychotherapist, counsellor and supervisor in Hammersmith, West London. He has an enduring interest in using myth, story and visual imagery as portals for understanding and unravelling the mysteries and challenges of existence. Counterbalancing his psychological work, Steve is a painter, printmaker and illustrator. Website: www.stevesimpson.org.uk. Email: stevesimpson_therapy@hotmail.co.uk.

MARK SKELDING Diploma in Psychosynthesis Counselling (NZ), Diploma in Psychosynthesis Psychotherapy (NZ), MNZAC, MPAnzA. Mark facilitates the Fundamentals and Foundation Year programmes for the Institute of Psychosynthesis NZ, has a private practice in Thames and Auckland, is a founding trustee of PAnzA (Psychosynthesis Aotearoa/NZ Australia), a Heart Politics convenor, and co-ordinator of T3-TransitionTownThames. Email: songlines@paradise.net.nz.

MOLLY YOUNG BROWN MA, combines psychosynthesis, ecopsychology, and Deep Ecology in her teaching, writing, coaching, and workshops. Publications include: *Unfolding Self: The Practice of Psychosynthesis*; *Growing Whole: Self-realization for the Great Turning*; and with Joanna Macy, *Coming Back to Life: Practices to Reconnect Our Lives, Our World*. Email: Molly@MollyYoungBrown.com. Websites: www.mollyyoungbrown.com, www.psychosynthesispress.com.

Printed in Dunstable, United Kingdom

91222519R00141